BIOETHICS AND POPULATION
The Choice of Life

Michel Schooyans

Father Schooyans, philosopher and theologian, is a member of the Pontifical Academy of Social Sciences, Consultor of the Pontifical Council "Justice and Peace," and of the Pontifical Council for the Family. After having taught for ten years at the Catholic University of São Paolo, he has just retired as professor of political philosophy, social morality and the ethics of demographic problems at the Catholic University of Louvain, Belgium.

Translated by Rev. John H. Miller, C.S.C., S.T.D.

Central Bureau, CCVA
3835 Westminster Place
St. Louis, Missouri

Printed by
St. Martin de Porres Lay Dominican Community
New Hope, Kentucky 40052

TABLE OF CONTENTS

17. A law that punishes abortion is odious for women and ignores their rights.

18. Is democracy possible with only a minimum of political morality?

19. Should not the liberalization of abortion be considered an important step in the long march toward the liberation of women?

20. Isn't the dignity of women better honored when their right to abort is recognized?

21. Doesn't the liberalization of abortion concern certain particular categories of women?

22. Despite everything, doesn't abortion afford a relief to women's distress?

23. When a woman's distress is extreme, cannot abortion, nevertheless, be considered a lesser evil?

24. What should one do when the life of mother and/or child is in danger?

25. Does promoting the advancement of women in society include preventing abortion?

Chapter IV: Rape   15

26. Is abortion justified in the case of rape?

27. Faced with so many rapes, abortion is a source of security for the woman.

28. Can we not see that one of the frequent causes of abortion in that the father will not assume responsibility for the child?

29. Don't exceptional situations, such as AIDS in Africa and rapes in the former Yugoslavia, justify exceptional measures?

Chapter V: Euthanasia   17

30. How does legalization of abortion open the way to legalization of euthanasia?

31. Some assert that we are easily sliding from abortion to euthanasia. Despite all, aren't we dealing with very different problems?

32. How could German society be led to organize mass extermination?

33. Did not economic factors reinforce the perverse influence of this irrational vitalism?

Chapter VI: The Body a Disposable Object   19

34. Would our law tend to accept a concept of the body regarded as a thing?

35. Can we point to examples showing that the body is treated as an object?

36. What are the consequences entailed by the questioning of the non-availability of the body?

37. Isn't the liberalization of abortion the consequence of a new perception of the human body?

38. Are we not quickly coming to consider the body as another thing among others?

39. Wasn't there, however, some reluctance on the part of pharmaceutical firms regarding their research on contraceptive products?

40. Law reflects morals. Since abortion has become part of our morals should it not be legalized.

41. Don't laws liberalizing abortion at least have the advantage of limiting these?

42. In a democracy it's the majority that decides; so parliament can change the law.

43. In order to protect itself, cannot society pass prohibitions?

44. Does not the failure to apply the law put to scorn a state based on law?

45. A "juridical void" is denounced in some countries. Is such a void not inadmissible?

46. Since people are having abortions, isn't it better to legalize them and make them a medical procedure so that they will be performed "under good conditions"?

47. Can we reproach legislators for defining the conditions under which abortion can be authorized?

48. The fact is that there are clandestine abortions. Hence, would it not be better to legalize abortion in order to diminish their number?

49. Haven't judges the power to make laws liberalizing abortion be respected?

50. Isn't there a difference between decriminalizing abortion, that is to say removing it from the penal code, and liberalizing it, that is to say making it easier and more free?

51. In the debates about liberalizing abortion, some have at times requested that the state remove the guilt of abortion. What does this term mean?

52. Has the practice of abortion changed the image of medicine?

53. Can one envisage a personality split among doctors?

54. Should we not fear the interference of morality in the scientific domain?

55. How can doctors be led to subordinate the interest of the individual to that of society?

56. Isn't the practice of abortion going to change the image of magistrates?

57. How will the attitude of judges who fail to pursue their duty impact on political society?

78. Isn't it shocking to suggest a parallel between the Nazi torturers and the abortionists of today?

79. What can one actually say about world population?

80. At least a fifth of humanity lives in a situation of absolute poverty, in subhuman conditions, unworthy of man. For the sake of these people and their families, would it not be better to prevent them from having children?

81. Won't it contribute to the happiness of the poor to have access to sterilization and abortion made easier?

82. Isn't a terrible threat hanging over humanity: the "demographic explosion" of the Third-World?

83. Some go so far as to speak of a "demographic bomb" all ready to explode.

84. Does this fear of population growth in the Third World involve certain countries in particular?

85. How is the demographic situation in Europe?

86. How has Europe come to such a demographic collapse?

87. Doesn't the United States also experience a demographic collapse comparable to that of Europe?

88. Would the demographic implosion in Europe be of such a nature to worry the United States?

89. Since the demographic situation of Europe is so grave, why are so few politicians concerned about it?

90. How is the problem of abortion presented in a country like Japan where it has become commonplace?

91. Has anyone an idea of the consequences of the collapse of fertility in the developed countries?

92. Hasn't mankind, by its very mass, become a nuisance for the environment?

93. There is often mention made of a campaign arising from the rich and powerful who devote themselves to limiting the world population of the poor in order to avoid the obligation of sharing their wealth. Isn't that a rather gloomy outlook for society and the future of the world?

94. Why is it that such publications are so poorly known?

95. Can facts be cited to support the contention that this campaign exists?

96. Is it in this context that the abortive pill RU 486 appears?

97. Would this mean that the specialized agencies of the United Nations and the United Nations itself are implicated in the anti-birth campaigns in the poor countries?

98. It is almost unthinkable that an institution of such prestige as the United Nations would offer support to the politics of demographic "containment" involving the practice of abortion.

99. Who will profit by this change?

100. Is this change profitable to certain particular nations?

101. Does the Kissinger Report speak of abortion?

102. Would there be a relationship between the demographic politics of the US and the change observed in the nature of the UN?

103. How can it be explained that the Western democracies join forces with the United States to curb the demographic growth of the Third World?

104. Is the attitude of these rich people shared by all the citizens of the US and the Western democracies?

105. Isn't it inconsistent for Western nations to export abortifacient products while continuing to pose as champions of democracy and development?

106. In the final analysis, who are really responsible for and are the real restorers of contemporary totalitarianism?

107. When all is said and done, if no action on behalf of human life is undertaken on a worldwide basis, isn't what is emerging a new war?

108. Isn't it excessive to speak of war in respect to abortion?

Chapter XIII: Prevention—Repression—Adoption

109. Isn't there at least one point on which partisans and adversaries of abortion are in accord?

110. Instead of repressing abortions, wouldn't it be better to prevent it?

111. Don't legislators who liberalize abortion have a preventive role?

112. Is it necessary, then, to maintain a repression of abortion?

113. Does adoption offer an "alternative" to abortion?

Chapter XIV: The Church and Childbearing

114. What does the Church say about abortion?

115. Regarding respect for human life and in particular respect for the life of the unborn, isn't it a fact that many Christians are in open opposition to the Church?

116. Do not some Christians run the risk of being reproached today with the same lack of courage as lamentable as that of some Christians of former times?

117. The Catholic Church should take into account the evolution of morals and adapt her conception of sin to them.

118. Why does the Church reject contraception?

119. Must we not carefully distinguish contraception through use of hormones from sterilization?

120. When you say responsible parenthood you say contraception. But the Church is opposed to contraception.

121. The Church makes it necessary for people to have recourse to abortion because she is opposed to contraception.

122. Isn't effective contraception the best way to avoid abortion?

123. What consequences are entailed by the separation of sex from procreation in the conjugal union?

124. In what way does the contraception practiced by some couples have a political dimension? Isn't it a purely private affair?

125. With her morality, doesn't the Church have a heavy responsibility for the world's demographic growth?

126. Why do so many reject the Church's message about misery in the Third World?

127. Doesn't the conjugal morality of the Church favor having children?

128. According to some specialists, the Church's position in the matter of contraception and demography is going to cause dramatic consequences — notably famine.

129. Why would one institute "permits to procreate" in wealthy countries where the birth rate is suffering such a disquieting decline?

130. Where do we find the Church's teaching on population? Isn't it contained in her pro-birth conjugal morality?

131. Doesn't the Church completely neglect the demographic problems when she proclaims her beautiful principles concerning development?

132. In this question of demography, aren't Catholic moralists in bad faith? In effect, they say that development entails a drop in the birth rate, but they hide the fact that this decline in the birth rate is obtained in the developed countries by methods condemned by the Church.

133. Isn't it dreaming to imagine that natural methods can be widely distributed and used?

134. Isn't it out of naïveté, if not a provocative spirit, on the part of Chiristians to advocate recourse to natural methods?

135. Discussions concerning natural methods refers us, then, to an in-depth reflection on human development?

136. What, then, is the heart of the Church's social teaching on demography?

137. Why do the ideologues of demographic security give so much attention to ecological problems?

138. Don't the decriminalization of abortion and its practical consequence, its liberalization, pose serious threats to our society?

139. Are we not witnessing the execution of a scientific program of social engineering?

140. With nearly six billion inhabitants haven't we reached the limits of the earth's capacity?

141. When all is said and done, must we not stop speaking of overpopulation?

142. Is the "culture of death" a characteristic of our century?

143. Instead of being part of the "culture of death," isn't genetic manipulation oriented to the service of life?

144. Can we foresee the consequences of these manipulations and the legislation attempting to legitimize them?

145. In many of the reasons given, aren't there special reasons that impel Christians to promote respect for life?

146. Finally, would human life be a sign of hope for all men?

PREFACE

Immediately upon leading Dante throught the gate of Hell, Virgil pointed to a sorry mass of humanity and uttered these words:

> We have come to the place where I told you that you would see the wretched people who have lost the good of the intellect.

Is losing the good of the intellect really so significant a deprivation? Dante tells us that it puts us in Hell. The modern world thinks it places us on the road to Utopia. If the intellect has an object — truth, according to the tradition — would that object not suffocate a person's individual liberty? If one must conform to an external yardstick, how can one become a truly free and creative individual? So reasons the modern world.

Fr. Schooyans agrees with Dante. But the modern world is saying, in effect, "it is good that the intellect has no objective good because it releases us to create our own good, through committees, for example, whereby we reveal how broad-minded and collegial we are."

Fr. Schooyans will not be deceived. He knows only too well and explains to us only too clearly that if ethics is disconnected from truth and becomes a purely procedural phenomenon, what eventuates is not more liberty, but the arbitrary domination of one group of people over another. It is the truth that makes us free, not the committee decisions of a power elite.

In 1931 in Italy, nearly 99% of university professors gave their allegiance to Mussolini. Intellectuals, in the main, have forsaken their vocation to discover the truth of things, and have opted, instead, to exploit anyone who threatens their security. The most comtemptible of all abuses in the modern world, Schooyans contends, is "the abuse of intellectual power, for it wounds man in his very intelligence in which he is most like God."

The modern world dissolves freedom from truth and gives us the antithesis of freedom, slavery. It deprives us of any objective good and thereby alienates each citizen from the good of his neighbor. By inflating individual liberty until it bursts, the world not only destroys freedom, but deprives us of truth, goodness, justice, and love. As Schooyans rightly observes: "Freedom is the ability to consent to values (like good or justice) which reason can discover; it is the capacity to open oneself to another, to love."

Schooyans' message is, at root, a hopeful one. To arrive at this root, however, requires trudging through several layers of highly organized and firmly encrusted lies. The "neo-liberal current " for Schooyans, can be properly understood only when "it is situated in the funeral cortege of totalitarian ideologies that the twentieth century wanted to deify." When State, Party, and Race assume priority over the person, justice, and truth, then the essence of the "population problem" becomes the existence of people itself. But the solution to the problem of poverty is not to kill the poor but to share our goods with them. Justice demands that we give priority to the person and place at his disposal the many truths reason can uncover about the nature of human life and the means of allowing it to grow and flourish in community. The problem we must attack is poverty, not population. Justice demands care and development, not contraception, sterilization, abortion, and euthanasia.

Schooyans' hard-hitting message is appreciably softened by his question and answer format. The conversational style of the book gives it a personal quality that the reader will appreciate in contrast to the impersonal aproaches that characterize the mindset of modern bureaucracies. Althought the world gives lip service to the importance of "dialogue," it has lost sight of the objective center of all true "dia-logue," which is the "logos."

Three virtues characterize *Bioethics and Population*, virtues that are rarely present in the same work. Ther are: erudition, integrity, and soundness. Schooyans' reading reflects a vast area of scholarly thought. His uncompromising integrity shines forth from every page. His soundness reveals how well he has balanced paradoxes, organized his thought, and appreciated the complexity of his subject matter. Fr. Schooyans has given us a *tour de force* that is as insightful as it is frightening.

At a time in history when references to the cultures of life and death are made with increasing frequency, Schooyans' book is particularly welcomed. On the other hand, some will find it controversial. Those who do, however, would find it most instructive if they realized that at the heart of Schooyans' ethics is nothing more inherently controversial than the Golden Rule. In doing unto others what one would have them to unto us, and in not doing unto them what we would not have them do unto us allows each off us to find his proper place in the commonwealth of humanity.

The ancient Greeks knew, realistically that a law must be more than a law — it must be *eunomos*, a good law. Similarly, we can say that a book must be more than just words — it must be *eulogia*, good words. Fr. Schooyans has given us some good words in the hope that we will convert them into good deeds.

Donald DeMarco
University of St. Jerome's College

FOREWORD

The major problem of the nineteenth century, on the moral, social, economic and political planes, was the undeserved misery of the working class, with which we must link colonial exploitation. The major problem of our time, on the same planes, is much more serious than that of the nineteenth century. It concerns the undeserved contempt that human life is the victim of everywhere in the world.

This problem has been clearly seen since the first half of the twentieth century. However, its extreme gravity appears above all with the world campaign seeking, not only to dry up the sources of life by making sterilization commonplace, but also by the legalization of abortion — and very soon, without doubt, of euthanasia too.

This taking over of life is presented as the sole satisfactory solution in a whole series of cases people have portrayed as painful or dramatic. However, as experience shows, this commandeering of life raises more problems than it tries to solve.

Among other instances, the trouble in the region of Chiapas in southern Mexico at the beginning of 1994 should have made even the most opaque blinders fall off. These events find their deepest cause in the injustice and inequalities that the Indians of the San Cristobal de las Casas region have experienced. And if the same causes run the risk of producing the same effects, we must hasten to prevent such outbursts by remedying the injustices and inequalities. The international campaigns for sterilization and abortion reveal, in those who sponsor them, a refusal to remedy these injustices and inequalities. Once the victims become aware of them, the revolt will spread like a trail of gun powder, and nothing will be able to halt the violence.

On the other hand, it is amazing to see how careful the Clinton administration is, after the fall of the Soviet bloc, to prevent the emergence of any actual or potential enemy. The demographic collapse that is striking all of western Europe — and to which liberalized abortion is obviously no stranger — must please the imperial appetites of the transatlantic fatherland. Unborn babies in Europe are subjected to a program of destruction even before they are able to emerge as rivals to an America obsessed with its security and expansion.

We have discussed these problems in detail in two works: *L'Enjeu politique de l'avortement* and *La dérive totalitaire du libéralisme*, and we will frequently refer to them. As a sequel to these two books, we propose a series of arguments especially for all those who need a practical instrument to use in the debates in which they take part.

And so we are going to examine here in simple terms some of the arguments advanced most often in the discussion about respect for life. These discussions touch on some fundamental questions of bioethics, but they will be examined in the light of actual demographic phenomena. This examination will carry us, then, well beyond the ins and outs of liberalizing abortion.

Epiphany 1994, Louvain-la-Neuve.

INTRODUCTION

In the question of abortion, do not Christians wish to impose their **1.**
morality on others?

Christians have no monopoly in the defense of human life. Respect for all human life is a fundamental precept of universal morality proclaimed by all great civilizations, and it is the warp and woof of every democratic society.[1] If this right to life is not respected and protected, all other rights are threatened (cf. 59). The exercise of freedom requires respect for the right to life. In Belgium, for example, the law of 1867 suppressing abortion was voted in under a homogeneous liberal government; at that time Christians were in the opposition.[2]

Do we have the data on the number of abortions in the world? **2.**

The data on this subject is actually more plentiful than twenty years ago, but it must always be gathered with care. This concerns, first of all, the difficulties of those who collect it. Moreover, according to the thesis to be proved, data can be inflated or diminished. In any case, the data is unverifiable up to a certain point.

According to the data of the World Health Organization (1990), there would have actually been between 40 and 60 million abortions every year in the world.[3] Even if these numbers are subject to question, it must make us reflect. Forty million, that is the approximate number of those who died in the Second World War. Forty million abortions each year, that is a massacre without precedent in history. It is at once a demographic and moral disaster.

EXPLANATION OF ENDNOTES:

We abbreviate the endnotes at the beginning in this way:

EPA refers to *L'enjeu politique de l'avortement* (Paris: Oeil, 1991);

DTL refers to *La dérive totalitaire du libéralisme* (Paris: Editions Universitaires, 1991).

—The reader will frequently find in the body of the text the indication (cf. + number): please refer then to that question number to complete the subject treated. For example, in the reply to the Question 1, (cf. 59) indicates that the reader will find at Question 59 a complement to reply 1.

—In the same way, the Index refers the reader to the Question numbers.

[1] Regarding democracy and the "golden rule," see EPA, pp. 99 ff., n. 19; 112; 198 and Chapter IV.

[2] Cf. EPA, p. 59, n. 4

[3] Cf. DTL, p. 75. See the three volumes prepared by the Department of Economic and Social Development of the United Nations, *Abortion Policies: A Global Review* (New York: U.N., 1992).

In the case of France, see, among others, the publications of l'Association pour recherche et l'information démographique (APRD), 12, rue Beccaria, 75012 Paris. In particular cf. the collection, *L'enjeu démographique*, 1981, especially pp. 44 ff. The same association published in 1979 *Dossier avortement: les vrais chiffres*, with an introduction by Gerard-François Dumont on "the duty of providing information" (pp.2 f.). The famous demographer has also published two articles on this problem: "Le nombre véritable des avortements. On ne doit pas déroger à la vérité des chiffres," *La Croix-l'Évènement*, March 3-4, 1991; and "Avortement, le refus de voir," *L'Homme Nouveau*, April 18, 1993.

In the case of England, see the study of R. Whelan cited at Question 41, note 3.

THE UNBORN CHILD

Is the unborn child a human being?   **3.**

Even the laws liberalizing abortion begin by declaring the human character of the being whose killing in certain cases they are nevertheless authorizing. Article I of the Veil-Pelletier Law in France displays typical incoherence in this regard: "The law guarantees respect for every human being from the beginning of life. This principle must not be breached except in the case of necessity according to conditions defined by this present law."[1] This procedure is sometimes called "tactic of dispensation": it declares a principle indisputable only to proceed immediately to enumerate the conditions or circumstances in which the law determines it doesn't apply. (cf. 31, 61, 65). We find this tactic regularly in the projects and legal propositions concerning euthanasia.

In the case of a conceived infant, it is precisely because it is a human being that they want to prevent its birth. They know that the being will soon be a baby, then an adolescent, then an adult. It is because it promises to be a baby, an adolescent, and an adult that they want to suppress it.

Why do certain supporters of abortion cast doubt on the human   **4.**
character of the unborn infant?

Men have cast doubt on the human character of certain beings whenever they sought arguments to exploit or exterminate their fellow human beings.[2]

In antiquity slaves were considered as things and barbarians as second class men.[3] In the sixteenth century, some conquerors considered the Indians as "beasts in human appearance." The Nazis looked upon some men as "non-men," as *Unmenschen*. To these arbitrary classifications dictated by the masters corresponded real discrimination and this, in turn, "legitimized" exploitation or extermination (cf. 32).

5. Does biological progress permit us to maintain any doubt about the human character of the infant before birth?

In veterinary medicine no one asks whether the embryo of a dog is animated with a feline, ovine or bovine life.

The product of human procreation is a human being. The human character of the embryo resulting from the union of man and woman has not been questioned except by those who wanted to fabricate premises to justify abortion or experimentation on embryos (cf. 69).

Moreover it is significant and indeed revealing that certain promoters of in vitro fertilization and transfer of the embryo say they are morally worried about the fate of those embryos remaining in vitro but not the ones transplanted in vivo.[4]

6. Is abortion justified when the conceived infant is not wanted?

a) We have no criterion at our disposal for saying whether a wanted child will be happy or whether an unwanted child will be poorly loved or unhappy. There are many unforeseen children who are well loved; there is no lack of wanted children who are unhappy. Child abusers *desire* children.

Furthermore, we must remark that, even if he or she is wanted, the child who survives always runs a risk, indeed innumerable risks, from his parents and from society. How can we forget that a child wanted before his birth can be perceived as undesirable once he is born, whether because of his development (delinquency, for example), or whether because of a change in his parents (disagreement, for example).

Education for acceptance is needed, then.

b) Let us add that in a few months of pregnancy, the mother's psychology changes almost always from vexation to acceptance, and from acceptance to love. The desire for a child isn't fixed at the stage when he takes form at the beginning of pregnancy; it progresses, it matures. Probably we were not all wanted; but we are sure that we were welcomed.

Moreover, the natural structure for acceptance of a child is the *united couple*, where two human beings constitute a *family*, that is to say, they form a project that involves duration, fidelity, trust, in order to face the unforeseen together (cf. 63). An entire climate has developed in society which, all too often, dissuades a couple from planning and procreating, or makes a couple that has children feel guilty.

7. Isn't the wanted child the fruit of responsible parenting?

The only parenting worthy of a man is responsible parenting (cf. 121). No one denies that. Some planning of births is necessary for all couples. But what does planning mean? Is it a matter of totally controlling fertility by any means whatsoever: radical contraception, remedial abortion, sterilization, euthanasia of handicapped infants. . .?

If fact, if we admit that we can eliminate all the undesired ones, human society will be destroyed. If we do not allow the presence of others with their differences, life in society becomes infernal. It was Sartre who said, "Hell is other people!"[5]

8. With the techniques of medically assisted procreation available, isn't it normal for parents to demand an infant of perfect quality?

The same kind of logic motivates people not to accept the infant unless it is wanted and not to want an infant unless it is of "perfect quality." In both cases, the infant isn't wanted for itself; it isn't wanted except insofar as it satisfies the couple's desire. If it is not wanted, news of its arrival thwarts the wishes of the couple. If it isn't perfect, the coming child doesn't respond to the expectations of the couple (cf. 122).

In both cases, the life of the child is in a sort of suspended sentence: its life or death are entirely at the discretion of those who want it.

9. How does the desire for a perfect infant lead to abortion?

When we accept as a principle that a being can be given existence *because* it is the object of desire, we necessarily say that a being can be deprived of existence *because* it is not the object of desire.

The unwanted infant can be eliminated for the sole reason that it is not desired. The child who doesn't conform to the qualities required can also be eliminated for the sole reason that he doesn't have the qualities required of him.

This explains the fact that the indications for abortion have a tendency to vary and multiply. The multiplication of "eugenic" or "orthogenic" indications for abortion are the corollary of a vision that reduces the infant to an object of desire.

10. We have become sensitive to the quality of life. Many conceived infants will be unhappy and will not have a life of quality. Abortion prevents this problem and solves it.

a) One may have reasons to think that the context in which the child will live is not favorable to the happiness of the child to be born. Faced with such a quandary, we have to ask ourselves which solution is the more humane: abort the infant or make an effort to create for him the best conditions of existence?

b) The proposition we have just examined rests on the following presupposition: *life isn't worth living unless one begins with a certain threshold of quality.* It is obvious that we are in the realm of complete subjectivity.[6] What is this quality of life, and where is its threshold found? What makes for the happiness of one will not do so for another, and Peter begins to smile at what makes Paul think of suicide.

c) If it is lawful to kill a human being because he risks being so poor that his life would no longer be worth living, then it is also legitimate to kill all those who are already dying of hunger. Evidently no one would dare support this consequence, as compulsory a logic as it holds. The flaw of such reasoning thus comes to the light of day: *the solution to poverty is, not to kill the poor man, but to share our goods with him* (cf. 136).

d) Our society has never been as rich as it is today. It will suffice to reach a political decision to give maternity aid that is well thought out, well applied, and well controlled so that every infant is born having at his disposal the material minimum required to assure a worthy existence for him or her.

11. In the name of having a right to a life of quality, should we not refuse life to a being for whom nothing but suffering or handicap is foreseen?

The greatest threat to health is the threat of losing life itself. We simply cannot identify human *life* and the *quality* of life (cf. 23). These two notions are not even on the same level, somewhat as democracy and the qualities (or defects) of democracy are not on the same level. We are in a democratic regime or we are, for example, in a totalitarian regime. The fact that one is in a democratic regime does not prevent such a regime from having defects. These defects must be combatted, but the worst way of rectifying them is to destroy the democracy itself (cf. 40, 59). Here we touch on the question examined in no. 42.

All the same, if an infant is handicapped or an old man is bedridden, they always live a human existence. Their infirmity brings no intrinsic modification to this basic given.

This means the rights of man are inherent in the human being *because* he lives a *human* existence. This human character is clearly inscribed in his body: human existence involves a corporeal dimension that is essential to it. To speak of the physical or psychological qualities of this man makes no sense except relative to this existence. *Relative to* means that we cannot speak of qualities except *in relationship to* a real existence, dependent on it.

When the awaited infant is affected by some malformation wouldn't   12.
it be better to have recourse to abortion in order to spare him a
life unworthy of a man?

a) This question takes up again a preceding one (cf.11). Faced with a handicap, what solution should we choose as the more humane: kill the infant or help him to lead the best life possible taking into consideration his abilities (cf. 15)? If the mother or family do not feel they have the strength to meet this situation, must society drive them into a corner with a desperate solution by leaving them to carry the full weight all alone, or, on the contrary, should it try to help them undertake it?[7]

b) The really tragic thing is that, in certain milieux, the infant is reduced to a consumer good: it is wanted if it gives pleasure (cf. 37). It's like a video or a car: if it pleases it is accepted; if not, it is aborted.

The infant affected by some malformation is nonetheless a member, entirely on its own, of the human species; it deserves to live like all other human beings. If we eliminate it because of its malformation, we will eliminate those who do not have the hoped-for color of skin or sex. In short, it isn't the handicapped child but the handicap that is not wanted.

c) Let us take the example of infants with Down's syndrome. What gives us the right to decide that they will be unhappy? If we ask their parents, we find that the overwhelming majority of them say that these children are happy: they ignore what causes problems for "normal" people! Moreover, most of these parents are happy with their child, also taken care of almost always by brothers and sisters (cf. 13). Children with Down's syndrome have also been the cause of the reconciliation of couples whose relationship was shaky.

Infants reduced to a *vegetative life* have been known to transform totally the life of their parents who, welcoming them with all their hearts, are now intent that no infant be rejected.

d) This question is also in line with the preceding one in the sense that one can wonder what makes an existence worthy of man. Certainly, there are tragic cases and lives whose meaning, from a human viewpoint, we have great difficulty in discerning. But isn't it very presumptuous to say that just because we cannot see it, the meaning is nonexistent? Doesn't that manifest an intellectual and moral decision whose conclusions cannot be rationally justified? And then where do you draw the line beyond which existence is unworthy of man? A woman in France agreed to an abortion because the infant she carried risked being sterile![8]

13. Prenatal diagnosis enables us to detect Down's Syndrome. With such scientific progress does one have the right to let live an infant who will be a cross for his parents and whose own life will never develop?

Do you know the celebrated bass Ruggero Raimundi? On November 23, 1989, he related an astonishing thing on Jacques Chancel's radio program.[9] Outside the theatre, Raimundi never sings. He makes but one exception: he sings for his fourth son, Rodrigo, "who was born with one too many chromosomes." Now, mama and papa and the three big brothers, accepted and welcomed this little Mongoloid. "For my wife and me, Rodrigo is now a gift from God. A gift from heaven. He has brought us to discover depths of soul within us we never suspected. Yes, treasures which in the normal circumstances of life we wouldn't have seen, because we ignore them." And with his artistic sensitivity, Raimundi added: "Still today, when people hear the word *Mongoloid* many of them think it is something to reject, not allow to be born, or to put in hospitals, special places. That is an appalling error. Mongoloid infants should be kept within the family circle. We must love them, surround them with affection. They return your love a hundredfold to the point of extravagance! You cannot imagine my happiness when I see Rodrigo again and sing for him. He is there, smiles at me and kisses me without end. It's indescribable. Rodrigo is very endearing, without doubt, because he feels himself accepted as he is."

[1] Cf. EPA, pp. 48, 53.

[2] On the human character of the unborn infant, see Jerome Lejeune, *L'enceinte concentrationnaire*, Paris: Fayard, 1990.

[3] Cf. DTL, p. 173.

[4] We have examined the moral problems posed by in vitro fertilization and transfer of the embryo in *Power over Life Leads to Domination of Mankind* (St. Louis: Central Bureau, 1996); see esp. Ch. III. See also Dr. Philippe Gauer, *Le choix de l'amour. Diagnostic anténatal* (Paris: Tequi, 1989). Benoît Bayle devoted his doctoral thesis in medicine (Paris, 1992) to *La destruction de l'embryon humain dans la société contemporaine*. After reviewing abortion, the IUD, contraception, female sterilization, medically assisted procreation, the author questions our "embryo-killing society" and proposes a "sexual counterrevolution" based on respect for the human embryo.

[5] *Huis clos.*

[6] Cf. EPA, Ch. IX.

[7] See the beautiful book of Jerome Lejeune and Geneviève Poullot, *Maternité sans frontières*, Paris: V.A.L., 1986.

[8] For an example see EPA, pp. 50 f., n. 9.

[9] Under the title "Pavane pour un enfant divin," Yvonne Somadossi devoted a magnificent report on this broadcast in *Le Soir* (Brussels), Dec. 20, 1989.

WOMAN, SPOUSE AND MOTHER

Isn't a woman master of her own body?   **14.**

    Except in regions in which slavery still exists, no human being can become the *property* of another (cf. 34), the object of another's right. Now the unborn infant is not an organ of its mother; it is a unique, distinct being, with its own genetic individuality. This unique being will pursue its own original development without any interruption of continuity. A woman may not dispose of the existence of this being in the way the Roman paterfamilias could dispose of his children at any given moment.[1]

    Hence we must clarify a precondition: we must know what kind of society we are heading toward, what kind of society we want to promote. Do we want a society that welcomes every human being from the moment its presence is discernible, or a society that restores the privilege and even the prerogative of masters to dispose of the life of others? This last kind of society would rest on foundations very different from those that inspire democratic societies (cf. 17, 42); in it one would have to admit that all human beings are not to be respected equally.

Once a woman has chosen to have an abortion, should we not respect   **15.**
the decision she has made?

    If someone comes to me and says that he wants to commit suicide, I can adopt one of two attitudes: I can assist him in carrying out his decision, or I can try to understand the problems that push this man to suicide, help him resolve them and then dissuade him from killing himself. Likewise in the case of one who has decided on an abortion. Once we agree to recognize it, we see that suicide, abortion — as well as euthanasia — have this in common: they are always a defeat. And a defeat we make every effort to avoid (cf. 109).

16. *The right to abort, the right for women to dispose freely of their bodies, isn't this an essential demand of feminism?*

The height of machismo is for men to ransack women's intelligence and will while inducing them to become an object for sexual consumption.[2]

a) Taken in by the same chauvinism, women are inclined to desire their "dematernalization," that is, the neutralization of their maternal inclination[3] by taking hormones and even by means of mutilation. Already in some places, the same thing is happening with sterilization as with hysterectomy in many countries of Africa and the Middle East: women who have been sterilized wind up pointing their finger at those who aren't!

b) Under pressure from the Neo-Malthusian movement, women of the twentieth century have renounced the "comparative advantage" they have enjoyed since the dawn of time in relationship to men. Indeed, ever since the world has been the world, women enjoyed the secret of fertility. During this century they have consented to being deprived of this privilege and of being *alienated from it*. They share the management of their fertility with men or they abandon the charge of controlling it to them.

17. *A law that punishes abortion is odious to women and ignores their rights.*

Laws restricting abortion do not in any way contest the rights of women; rather they emphasize the right to life of the conceived infant, a right which people are trying to skirt around today. What these laws affirm is that no one may dispose of the life of an innocent (cf. 60). These laws simply put into practice a general principle of every democratic society: the equality of all human beings in the right to life. Hence, the penal character of these laws is but the consequence of an anterior, inalienable right of the unborn infant. It is the violation of this right that calls for and justifies a penal sanction.

18. *Is democracy possible only with a minimum of political morality?*

In every society, people must know what favors and what obstructs living together. Dishonesty is an obstacle in a good society; we must say the same of rape. This is also true of murder, especially when the victim cannot defend himself. Law cannot prevent the transgression, but it punishes it, and punish it it must. In a democratic society there may be circumstances that attenuate or aggravate murder or rape, but no one has the *right* to rape or to kill an innocent person. Abortion cannot be considered a woman's *right*. Rape and murder do not *become* crimes or offenses because the law says so. The law punishes[4] them because they *are odious*.

Should not the liberalization of abortion be considered an important   **19.**
step in the long march toward the liberation of women?

a) Along with unborn infants, the real victims of abortion are women, murdered in body and soul; the great beneficiaries of abortion are men and those who make a financial or other kind of profit from these operations[5]. The demand for the liberalization of abortion, or even freedom to have them, puts in dramatic light the phallic tendencies of our society (cf. 27).

b) This demand shows once again that women can make themselves objective accomplices of the very men who contrive to exploit them. In effect, it is a frightful paradox that women allow themselves to be associated with this demand. Indeed, it is men who insidiously insist on the supposed *rights* of women, all the while seeking to retain over them their uncaring domination.

Isn't the dignity of women better honored when their right to abort   **20.**
is recognized?

Liberalization of abortion marks a serious regression in women's patient pursuit of the recognition of their dignity.

Thanks to this liberalization:

—men create the conditions permitting them to dispose of any woman whatsoever, whenever they wish at their convenience;

—even in principle they relieve themselves of all responsibility toward the child they have begotten;

—they dispense themselves from promoting measures that would ameliorate the situation of women in society;

—women become exploitable objects to whom, sometimes sterilization is offered as a bonus or imposed;

—enflamed largely by the media, a conflict among work, sexual indulgence, leisure and maternity is exacerbated in them.

Doesn't the liberalization of abortion concern certain particular   **21.**
categories of women?

Studies undertaken in France and England show that it is above all single women, and adolescents in particular, who resort to abortion.

a) In England, in 1978, 65% of women who had abortions were celibate, widowed, divorced or separated. And this phenomenon is not peculiar to England; the same is found in France.[6]

11

b) Experience shows how, in particular, liberalization of abortion ravages adolescents, who, from the onset of womanhood, are delivered without defense to every exploitation, degradation and humiliation.[7] In 1978, in England, 2.6% of women who had abortions were less than sixteen years old.

c) Reflection on liberalizing abortion reveals, not only the vulnerability of the infant, but more so the extreme vulnerability of woman in society. As a consequence, it is urgent not to separate in our discussions the *integral* advancement of woman *and* the protection of the infant to be born.

22. *Despite everything, doesn't abortion afford a relief to women's distress?*

Set apart the appalling case of women who sacrifice their infant because they consider it an obstacle to their career, their vacations or their pleasure, future mothers in distress await our help and not that we kill their infant. Besides, it is not by killing an unborn infant that a woman's distressful situation is attenuated (cf. 28). The majority of women who abort are single. The enquiry already cited above, made in England, reveals that 65% of women having aborted were legally celibate (cf. 21). Does abortion resolve the problem of their solitude? In the end, on the contrary, doesn't it aggravate it? We must take into account that liberalized abortion relieves society of the duty of helping a woman in difficulty. Dramatically, this will merely support the ripping of her body and soul; she will be sent back again to her solitude more bruised than before. For — to say nothing of remorse — there is a kind of "short" distress, that inclines one to consider aborting, and a "long" distress, that keeps echoing after an abortion.

And so, before any other consideration, there are certain measures to take in order to help women in difficulty and to reassure women who find themselves pregnant: a discreet, effective and warm "companionship." In this way they can bring their pregnancy to term in the best possible conditions, with the prospect of confiding their infant to adoptive parents, if they so wish (cf. 111, 113). In short, one of the dramas of the present world is that there are too many children without parents and too many parents without children (cf. 124).

23. *When a woman's distress is extreme, cannot abortion, nevertheless, be considered a lesser evil?*

a) Common morality and good sense have a maxim that between two *unavoidable* evils, one must choose the lesser evil, and that the end does not justify the means, that is to say, one may never do evil so that good will result from it (cf. 24). This simple maxim is certainly applicable here. One cannot kill an infant with the hope of ameliorating the situation of its mother or of society.

b) Neither does the argument that there would be a *conflict of values* here apply. Life is, in effect, the first of all goods, the first of all values that is the pre-condition of one's access to all others (cf. 11). The infant's right to life precedes all the rights that its mother has relative to other values.[8]

What should one do when the life of mother and/or child is in danger? **24.**

This deals with a problem that, happily, has become most rare in practice. Nonetheless questions about this are very frequent. To what principles can we refer?

a) A good intention does not suffice to change the value of a moral act. More simply: the end does not justify the means. Thus one may not execute an innocent person in order to save the country. To save the Fatherland is a good end, but the goodness of the end does not justify sacrificing an innocent person. Nor do circumstances change the moral value of an act. They can only attenuate or aggravate the responsibility of the agent.

b) The principle for solving this question is simple: one does not choose between the life of the mother and that of the child. One may not sacrifice an innocent life for another. Nevertheless, while doing everything possible to save the mother and preserve the life of the infant, the latter can perish due to the intervention. We desire above all to save both, but in doing everything that is humanly possible, it can happen that we end up with a consequence we did not desire: the death of the infant.

c) To *desire* to provoke the death, even indirectly, of an innocent person can never be licit even for a good end, for example saving the mother. It can happen that an action, even a good one like caring for the mother with cancer, entails an unfortunate consequence, neither willed nor desired, in the death of the infant the mother carries.

d) To sum up, it can happen that in trying loyally to save either one, the other becomes a victim. We are in the presence of a similar situation when one searches for victims of a cave-in. What one wishes to do is, first of all, to save everyone who can be saved.

Whenever one performs an act with a double effect, one positive, the other negative, one never wills the negative effect; one is resigned to it: one doesn't desire it; he tolerates it (cf. 23).

25. *Does promoting the advancement of women in society include preventing abortion?*

The woman is the one who is the first to recognize in her body the presence of a new human being. She is the first to be invited to welcome it freely. She is the first to propose that others also welcome it.[9]

To promote the dignity of women is then also to restore the value of the mother's irreplaceable role in society. Instead of blaming those who have children, or of spending oneself in byzantine discussions about the existence or non-existence of the maternal instinct, we have to create the conditions in which women really have the possibility of being mothers, even if they do not want to or cannot give up their profession.

[1] Cf. EPA, P. 53.
[2] Cf. EPA, pp. 124-126.
[3] *Idem*.
[4] Cf. EPA, pp. 32 f.; 45 f.; 87.
[5] Cf. EPA, p. 41, n. 8. Regarding the traumatic effects of abortion, see Susan M. Stanford, Une femme blessée, Paris: Fayard, 1989.
[6] Cf. EPA, p. 19.
[7] Cf. EPA, P. 19 and Ch. XIII.
[8] Cf. EPA, Chs. II and IV.
[9] Cf. Marie Hendrickx, "Quelle mission pour la femme?" *Louvain* (Louvain-la-Neuve) n. 4 April 1989, pp. 15 f; See also EPA, P. 120, N. 4.

RAPE

Is abortion justified in the case of rape? **26.**

Can we remedy a grave injustice by committing a still more grave injustice?

The violated woman must be better defended by judicial authority; it ought to find ways of dissuading prospective rapists from their activity. On the other hand, abortion brings about behavior hardly respectful of the woman and by that fact is conducive to making rape more commonplace (cf. 27 f.).

Faced with so many rapes, abortion is a source of security for the **27.**
woman.

In 1990 there were 100,000 rapes in the United States. That represents a 6% increase over the preceding year and 12 rapes an hour. Liberalization of abortion creates a violent mentality in which the stronger has right on his side and the weaker cannot resist the stronger. By that very fact, it leads to making rape commonplace. Hence, in a general way, such liberalization inevitably tends to expose women more and more to the ascendancy of men, the principal beneficiary of such legislation (cf. 19).

We can also cite the story of a young woman who arrived in Belgium without much money. Before leaving her native country, she had been raped. She found that she was pregnant and decided to keep the child. The rapist was still at large. Now many years later, this woman met the man in her life; she married him and he adopted the child, though he was not its father. Since then, the happy couple had several children.

Can we not see that one of the frequent causes of abortion in that the **28.**
father will not assume responsibility for the child?

This fact sets in relief a certain masculine cowardliness as well as the discriminatory complacency of the law regarding men. Yes, it's true; generally, one of the frequent causes of abortion is that the father refuses to assume responsibility for the child (cf. 19, 27).

Is that a reason for encouraging women to have an abortion? The law, which should protect that infant, must equally protect its mother and every woman. Women in difficulty don't expect us to suppress the infant but to help them (cf. 22). We can contribute toward making every maternity a source of great joy by our attitude of welcome.

29. *Don't exceptional situations, such as AIDS in Africa and rapes in the former Yugoslavia, justify exceptional measures?*

It's much the same in the matter of rape as in the matter of AIDS. The fight against AIDS with its publicity all over the place for a preventative serves causes other than that of health[1]. The one suffering from AIDS is sometimes considered less as a person needing care than as someone whom others use to join another battle. The stake in this battle is massive shamelessness of youth which is abused physically and psychologically; it's the transformation of the world into an immense brothel.

The same goes for rape. Just as we recently saw on the occasion of the rapes committed in ancient Yugoslavia, the fight against rape serves causes other than the violated women. The victims of rape are regarded less as persons who must be helped than as beings used to impose abortion as commonplace.

In both cases, they insist that "we don't have a choice": here we have a "situation of distress"' there a "situation of urgency." Freedom, we are assured, has no place here: we must bow before percentages and situations. These situations are so pressing that suddenly everything is permitted.

[1] See our article, "Jean-Paul II et le sida," (AIDS) in *Famille chrétienne* no. 801 (May 20, 1993) 14-16.

EUTHANASIA

How does legalization of abortion open the way to legalization of **30.**
    euthanasia?

  The conception of human life that inspires promoters of euthanasia is fundamentally the same as for promoters of abortion. Both believe my life and that of others makes no sense except for pleasure, interest or utility (cf. 15). If another is an obstacle to my enjoyment, if he is useless to me, I can do away with him if another cannot live a life of pleasure, his life can be suppressed (cf. 142).

  This last remark shows that there is a real link between eugenics (today euphemistically called *orthogenics*) and euthanasia: whether it is a question of an infant or an older sick person, their existence is not admissible unless they don't bother us or if they can enjoy pleasure.

  Therein we see that a hedonist society, one which maximizes the search for pleasure, fatally degenerates into a society of violence and death (cf. 34-39; 142 f.).

Some assert that we are easily sliding from abortion to euthanasia. **31.**
    Despite all, aren't we dealing with very different problems?

  a) We must insist on a fact: in countries in which abortion has been legalized, there rapidly arose projects or proposals to make laws authorizing euthanasia. Moreover, among those who fight for euthanasia, we also find people who fight for abortion.[1]

  b) We also know that in order to legalize abortion, people almost always began by breaking the law and defying the judges — all that in order to change the law. The tactic of *fait accompli* is also found in the case of euthanasia: they engage in it in order to legalize it eventually. This process of legalization follows a proven schema. At first timidly expressed, combatted, lost sight of, revised proposals surface with implacable insistence. Little by little they tame public opinion and bring the reluctance of legislators to an end.[2] They often finish by "triumphing" thanks to the "tactic of dispensation" (cf. 3, 65).

c) Contemporary history shows us also that the promoters of euthanasia have sometimes used another route to achieve their end. Nazi Germany, for example, had regulated abortion; it facilitated it for the so-called impure races but opposed it for the Aryan race. But it was above all sterilization on a grand scale that prepared minds to allow euthanasia (cf. 137).

32. How could German society be led to organize mass extermination?

In Germany the Nazi ideology had been prepared by theorists' exaltation of the Aryan race's superiority. This so-called superiority, of the biological order essentially, presented the race as one of masters (cf. 69). This superior race, with the superman which characterized it, is beyond good and evil in morality.

Here we are dealing with an *irrational vitalism* whose inevitable corollary is *nihilism* and the fascination with death (cf. 142 f.). The whole of society is organized to serve the protection of the race's purity, always threatened with degeneration by the weak (cf. 55). Starting from that point Hitler's Germany organized the sterilizations, abortion, euthanasia as well as the "final solution" according to discriminatory criteria.

33. Did not economic factors reinforce the perverse influence of this irrational vitalism?

After the First World War, Hindenburg instituted in Germany an obligatory, strictly regulated economy. The application of this regulation was entrusted to a network of omnipresent bureaucrats.

It was notably by this means that the General opened the way to Hitler, whose thought, moreover, was steeped in irrational vitalism. Named chancellor by Hindenburg in 1933, Hitler found at his disposal a bureaucratic apparatus put in place precisely to rule the economy. And, profiting from the organization controlling economic life, he had no difficulty in controlling all of society.

[1] Cf. EPA, 42; 96; 206.
[2] Cf. *ibid*. 14 f.; 57; Ch. VIII.

THE BODY
A DISPOSABLE OBJECT

Would our law tend to accept a concept of the body regarded as a thing? **34.**
Speaking historically, our law reached a decisive step when it began to consider the human person as an unbreakable, indivisible unity, and in consequence the human body was not a disposable thing. This non-disposability means that the body cannot be made the object of a contract, a transaction, a sale or be made an instrument.

Awareness of the non-disposability of the body nourished movements fighting for the abolition of slavery.[1] We also rightly consider regulation of slavery just plain nonsense.

We also find awareness of the non-disposability of the human body at the root of opposition to White slave trade. Again it is this awareness that, since the 19th century, is the source of the vindication for workers' rights to better working conditions: the laborer is not a machine. It is this same awareness that is particularly affirmed in some feminist movements combatting the myth of woman as an object.

Nevertheless, it is precisely this distinction between the world of men and the world of things that some are actually calling into question. Such questioning is the fatal price of a narrow concept of freedom that reduces the body to an object of pleasure (cf. 61).

Such questioning also results from the practices of which technological thinking boasts. In effect, many of these practices clearly *treat as objects*, not simply tissues and organs of the body, but *bodies themselves*.

Can we point to examples showing that the body is treated as an object? **35.**
Four examples will suffice to illustrate the practices that attack the non-disposability of the body.

First of all *in vitro fertilization and transfer of the embryo* (cf. 5), during which the embryo may be donated, sold, submitted to experimentation, or destroyed.[2] In addition, we also have the *donor baby*: an infant is conceived in order to be able to remove from it some cells which will be grafted on another.[3] Besides donor babies, we also have *surrogate mothers* who agree to put their own bodies at the disposition of a tenant and to deliver, on the date of maturity, another body, the one of which they were the carriers—all this on the basis of certain contractual conditions relative to bodies as though they were things.

As for abortion, it consists also in disposing of a body at someone's discretion as one would dispose of any object.

From all the evidence, the principle of the non-disposability of the human body is today seriously demolished in theory and practice.[4]

36. *What are the consequences entailed by the questioning of the non-disposability of the body?*

To the extent that this principle is disputed, even rejected, the road is opened wide to new forms of slavery.[5] The infant is considered a "piece of property" (cf. 12, 97) to which someone has a right, even the right of life or death (cf. 14). The poor can be "cannibalized," that is considered as breeding ground for organ transplants; their "fresh" organs become marketed objects. In exchange for a certain price, the poor man is separated from an organ of his body: he alienates it; he is alienated from it; in it he is alienated.

Finally, one assists even at making *livestock* out of the human population. Too many bodies harm the *ecological equilibrium*, and one must set quotas to their number to prevent them from becoming excessive and cause a deterioration in the surrounding milieu (cf. 137). We are told that economic laws must be respected and thus avoid that men, become too numerous, do not disturb the good functioning of the market.

In brief, an entire dynamic is set in motion. Since these things that are bodies are not persons, they can be disposed of before as well as after birth. The management of human livestock must obey the same rules that apply to the management of other material goods.

37. *Isn't the liberalization of abortion the consequence of a new perception of the human body?*

A narrow conception of freedom (cf. 61) without fail opens the way to an impoverished conception of the body. Despite appearances, we are witnessing a devaluing of the latter. And this devaluing is very perceptible in the phenomenon of *cannibalization*: one looks upon the human body as a reservoir of organs that can be removed for grafting.[6] Once severed from the person, the body becomes the seat of amorality. Corporeity is no longer perceived as a dimension of personality thanks to which man is situated in the world and time, and thanks to which he enters into interpersonal relationships with other subjects.

This is particularly apparent sexual behavior. The body is reduced to an object of individual pleasure. The sexual relationship becomes commonplace *because* it is depersonalized and is simply a source of pleasure. Now as this relationship is depersonalized, the partners become interchangeable. What counts is the variety and variation of pleasures. Individual reason, which calculates and compares the pleasures, is called upon to put to work the techniques that best serve to satisfy them.

The infant itself is perceived along the lines of an arithmetic of pleasures (cf. 12). It is seen either as a bothersome body to which abortion quickly puts an end, or as an object giving pleasure to the partners, or even as giving pleasure to only one of them.

Are we not quickly coming to consider the body as another thing   **38.** *among others?*

A depersonalizing conception of the body inevitably leads to a commercial exploitation of it.

Direct or indirect exploitation of individual sexual pleasures has become a powerful stimulant of economic, scientific and technological activity. This is evident for contraception and abortion over which specialized lobbies and even the Mafia jealously stand guard.[7] According to the United Nations Fund for Population, perfecting of a new product, before marketing, requires an investment in the range of $200,000,000.00.[8] That gives us an idea of the interests that are in play.

That clarifies also the reasons why the maximum extension of marketing contraception and contragestion is called for (cf. 122). All the potential customers are far from having become effective consumers, and passing from the first to the second category will be facilitated by the promotion of a hedonist morality, permissiveness in morals, pornography, initiation in licentiousness under the pretext of sex education. In turn, this promotion will contribute to the early spread of sexually transmitted diseases. Now, if these produce a large and defenseless clientele for pharmaceutical firms, they also create terrible dramas for individuals and families, and they weigh very heavily on the budget of the whole of society. And so, youth is doomed to depravity by companies with a cynicism bordering on madness, and scientific research as well as Social Security are powerless before the scope of the problem.

This is, then, fundamentally the same logic which, starting with a narrow concept of human freedom, ends by thinking that the human body can be disposed of as one disposes of a thing. The body is an *object* of alienation. An elementary truth is forgotten, namely, that it is not enough to say that we *have* a body, but one must say that we *are* a body. The whole of anthropology is certainly not exhausted by this formula, but it does affirm something essential.

39. *Wasn't there, however, some reluctance on the part of pharmaceutical firms regarding their research on contraceptive products?*

In a book that appeared in 1979, Carl Djerassi explains that pressure brought to bear by consumers unhappy with the harmful effects of contraceptive products, ran the risk of discouraging the firms' making these products.[9] These same firms also showed reluctance about the research leading to the production of new contraceptive preparations.

The author's analysis is all the more interesting in that it shows that the intervention of public powers became indispensable if they wanted to overcome the impasse created by the private firms' reluctance. With an unusual insistence, "demographic problems" were invoked (cf. 82), and they drew from that the argument that public powers must intervene (cf. 97 f.).

The"contraceptive establishment" was able to find a bypass thanks to the firm of Roussel-Uclaf (cf. 77), which benefitted from the support of the socialist government of France in order to produce the abortifacient pill RU 486, equally sponsored by WHO (Cf. 77).

This understanding between the public powers and the famous Germanic-French multinational learned a lot from the difficulties endured by the North American pharmaceutical companies. It shows how seriously can be taken threats of boycott that harass firms producing contraceptive drugs.

[1] These reflections owe much to Vincent Bourguet, "Penser esclavage aujourd'hui," *France Catholique* n. 2328 (Nov. 8, 1991) 23-25.

[2] On this problem see our book, *Power over Life Leads to Domination of Mankind* (St. Louis, Mo.: Central Bureau, CCVA, 1996) esp. Ch. III.

[3] See *Le Monde*, Feb. 18-19, 1990 and June 6, 1991; *Le Libre Belgique* of July 8, 1991.

[4]. Cf. Jean-Louis Baudouin and Catherine Labrusse-Riou, *Produire l'homme: de quel droit? Etude juridique et éthique des procréations artificielles* (Paris: PUF, 1987), esp. 185-210: "Du droit des personnes au droit des biens."

[5]. For a detailed analysis see DTL, esp. 147-156; 173-178 and passim.

[6] See DTL 122 ff.

[7] Cf. EPA 41.

[8] Cf. DTL 69.

[9] Cf. Carl Djerassi, *The Politics of Contraception* (New York and London: Norton, 1979).

VII

LEGISLATION

Law reflects morals. Since abortion has become part of our morals **40.**
    should it not be legalized.

One thing is certain in this matter: morals follow the law: "In modifying it," claims Simone Veil, "you can change the pattern of human behavior."[1] The best observers are in accord in recognizing that in France many of the women who undergo abortion would have *found another solution* had it not been for liberalized abortion laws (cf. 49). A democratic state recognizes the rights of its members to life, liberty and the security of their property. Such a state does not arrogate to itself the prerogative of declaring who, among the innocent, has the right to live or can be put to death. Nor does it arrogate the right to define who has the right to steal, to rape, or to kill. The state that would act in such a way would lose its democratic quality, for to integrate into law such infractions could not but favor the multiplication of the same infractions to the detriment of persons and property. But such is the fragility of democracy that it can even make for itself laws that put its own existence in peril.[2]

To enter on this path can lead very far indeed, for whenever one allows the elimination of unborn infants, one will quickly allow (it is allowed already) the death of the abnormal newborn, the incurably sick, the elderly — "all of them a burden to society."

Don't laws liberalizing abortion at least have the advantage of **41.**
    limiting these?

a) What is truly serious is the fact that there are abortions, with or without law, no matter how numerous. Laws liberalizing abortion aggravate this situation (cf.111), for people spontaneously expect that law responds to a demand of justice, that it not be in opposition to a fundamental principle of morality, such as the respect due to life. Besides, laws liberalizing abortion incite to abortion, anticipate it, make it commonplace, and make it become normal practice.[3]

b) Furthermore, these laws are the most disastrous of the whole history of humanity, and that for two reasons at least:

1) They create a juridical space for crime.

2) They corrupt youth by making it impossible for the young to distinguish good from evil and by destroying in them the most elementary sense of justice.

42. *In a democracy it's the majority that decides; so parliament can change the law.*

It is surely inexact to say that democracy is defined essentially by the mechanical and blind application of the rule of the majority. In 1931 in Italy nearly 99% of university professors gave their allegiance to Mussolini. And Hitler had been consecrated by parliamentary route.

It is also altogether inexact to pretend that democracy is a society in which anyone can do as he wishes and in which freedom can become license. Slaves had total sexual "liberty" in their huts.

What is characteristic of democracy is *anterior to the concept of majority rule* as the basis for the functioning of a regime of this type. Still, democracy is not characterized *first* by the way societies function. In the modern sense of the work, democracy is essentially defined by a *fundamental consensus* on the part of the whole social body regarding the *right of every man to live and to live with dignity.* It is primarily this right that must be promoted and protected (cf.61, 62). Consequently, it is the need for this protection that justifies the legislator's repression of the activity of individuals who would arrogate to themselves the "right" to dispose of life, liberty or the property of others.[4]

When consensus about this fundamental right is weakened, we risk returning to the privileges, to the injustices and cruelties of the Iron Age. The door opens to barbarism. The major illusion of Westerners is to think that since they have sat on all the contemporary forms of barbarism, they are definitively vaccinated against their triumphant return.

43. *In order to protect itself cannot society pass prohibitions?*

We must remark that a prohibition is never just the negative side of a positive will to protect a value or weaker individuals. The prohibition of stealing is the reverse side of the will to protect the property of others.

In every society one must know what are transgressions or risk returning to the jungle. There must be prohibitions, barriers

24

and they must be made known. The warning signals must be illuminated. Men being what they are, these prohibitions will without doubt be violated, but men will know that they are acting against a good, that they are infringing on a good (cf.117).

What is perverse about the liberalization and decriminalizing of abortion is that positive law suppresses the barriers. More seriously still is that transgression is presented as a right — even as good (legitimate) (cf.18).

It follows that entire categories of human beings are withdrawn from the protection of the law. Does that augur well for society in the future?

Does not the failure to apply the law show contempt for a state based on law?   **44.**

In order for there to be a state based on law in a country, it does not suffice that there be just any kind of legislation and that it be applied. Already for the Greeks that kind of law was not enough. They wanted *eunomos*: a law has to be good.

It can happen that law guarantees tyranny and legalizes despotism. Because China has its laws and they are applied doesn't mean that the Chinese live in a state based on law. A state based on law exists when the law is at the service of *justice for all* and not for the stronger or more numerous group.[5] If I expect the law to protect my life and liberty, it must also protect the life and liberty of others, especially of the weakest members of society.

A "juridical void" is denounced in some countries. Is such a void not inadmissible?   **45.**

Where there exists a law forbidding abortion, some magistrates, sometimes under pressure, hesitate to apply it. There is then a *judicial* void, for the law is not applied. This is not a *juridical* void, since the law exists.

This judicial void entails two consequences. On the one hand, it deprives the unborn infant of legal protection to which it has a right (cf.43). On the other hand, it fails to protect women faced with the customary impunity of man (cf.27) and all those who have an interest in inciting them to abort.[6]

Since people are having abortions, isn't it better to legalize them and make them a medical procedure so that they will be performed "under good conditions"?   **46.**

A medical procedure isn't defined by the use of instruments, medications and clinical installations, nor by putting knowledge and techniques to work, nor even necessarily the

25

abortionist's having a university diploma. A medical procedure is defined by its *finality*: to save life, to improve health. The giving of artificial respiration to a drowning victim is performing a medical procedure. The doctor who collaborates in torture does not perform a medical procedure. Just because the hangman's job is followed by an action of a doctor doesn't give the execution the quality of a medical procedure.

Likewise, just because abortion is done by a doctor and that the techniques used have been perfected, that is not enough to make an abortion a medical procedure.[7] From the club to the neutron bomb, men have not ceased to make "progress" in the art of killing their fellow human beings "under good conditions" (cf.53). In 1941, the Auschwitz doctors congratulated themselves on having "humanized" the manner of extermination in their camps: they had replaced carbon monoxide with a cyanide gas (cf.77). Rapes and murders always take place under bad conditions (at least for their victims). Are we going to organize centers in which rapes and murders would be performed under "good" conditions (for those who perform them), under medical supervision?

47. *Can we reproach legislators for defining the conditions under which abortion can be authorized?*

Liberalizing abortion is always, by that very fact, to regulate putting infants to death. To make work what the legislator decides, he will have to envisage well the forms of this funeral ceremony. Defining such forms will not be able to hide the decision always prior to proceeding to the execution of the innocent.

Hence, it would be absurd to imagine that regulation of abortion could retroactively legitimize abortion itself.

48. *The fact is that there are clandestine abortions. Hence, would it not be better to legalize abortion in order to diminish their number?*

a) It is certain that the number of clandestine abortions has been inflated precisely to instill fear and to change the law. How do we know that?[8]

—By the declarations made by doctors who have performed abortions. Bernard Nathanson, for example, estimates that the number of clandestine abortions in the USA has been considerably exaggerated.[9]

—By noting the effect of the law on the rate of births which falls after legislation.[10]

b) The French experience — alongside that of other countries in which abortion had been liberalized — shows that the

Veil-Pelletier law did not make abortions disappear, discreetly said not to be part of a "census." According to some estimates, these would be almost as numerous as those included in the count. All of which is to say that their number has not decreased.

Establishing an abortion mentality inevitably incites women to have it performed for motives and at times not anticipated by the law (cf.51), thus clandestinely and "under bad conditions."[11] That is easily understood: since in a democracy to forbid something without imposing a sanction makes no sense, decriminalizing inevitably contributes toward creating an abortion mentality that multiplies abortions both legal *and* clandestine. In this way the Soviet Union sometimes had more abortions than births.

Haven't judges the power to get respect for laws liberalizing abortion?　　**49.**

As experience demonstrates, the application of laws liberalizing abortion is practically uncontrollable;[12] it is all the more necessary to maintain legislation that is preventive, dissuasive and even repressive:

—preventive, for it must prevent an irreparable aggression against a human life exposed to being eliminated by someone stronger;

—dissuasive, for it must dissuade the mother from making the decision to abort and offer her alternative solutions that are warm and effective;

—repressive, for in a democratic society every attack on the freedom of another, and for greater reason on his life, must be sanctioned, while eventually taking into account attenuating or aggravating circumstances.

Isn't there a difference between decriminalizing abortion, that is to say　　**50.**
removing it from the penal code, and liberalizing it, that is to
say making it easier to obtain?

The distinction between decriminalizing and liberalizing abortion is very precarious.[13] To decriminalize means that abortion escapes penal sanction, which does not mean inevitably that it is permitted. Some analogous cases, of a lesser order it is true, are known: one does not punish the theft of bread committed by a starving poor person; one does not thereby declare that it is permitted. But in a democratic society in which so to speak whatever is not forbidden is permitted, to decriminalize abortion means to declare it unpunishable, which is the practical equivalent of authorizing it, liberalizing it, that is to connect it again as a right to individual liberties. To decriminalize abortion means to accept it, acknowledge it an established right; it is to legalize it, covering it with the authority of law. Hence, it means to deprive the unborn infant of all legal protection concerning his very existence — criminalizing abortion is but the logical consequence of such protection (cf.17, 43-35).

It is clear: the end envisaged is liberalization: to allow easy access to abortion. The means employed is decriminalization: promulgating a law authorizing abortion.

51. *In the debates about liberalizing abortion, some have at times requested that the state remove the guilt of abortion. What does this term mean?*

Not content to have the state legalize abortion, some expect the state to remove the guilt of abortion, that is to lift from it all connotation of a fault.

a) The very word used reveals that people perceive in a confused way that the state, as it is conceived in our civilization, goes beyond the mission conferred on it when it liberalizes abortion. Hence, they do not hesitate to request of this same state an intervention which implies, not only an increase of its powers, but a profound change in its very nature. When its own citizens ask the state to say what is right and what is evil, to say who can live and who can be eliminated, that state is pushed toward a totalitarian drift.[14] Here censure hits, not only the expression of the truth, but the truth itself.

b) They are establishing a new stereotyped language. It is the triumph of ideological discourse, and all reality and behavior must bend to it. One may not believe such discourse, but he acts according to it. This new language produces a perversion of reason and of moral conscience which entails, in turn, the destruction of the sense of justice (cf.41).

[1] *Times*, March 3, 1975.
[2] Cf. EPA 34; 55; 99 ff.
[3] Cf. EPA 34; 57. On this matter see the statistical study, unique of its kind, edited by Robert Whelan, with an introduction by Hubert Campbell, *Legal Abortion Examined. 21 years of Abortion Statistics.* London: Spuc Educational Research Trust, 1992.
[4] Cf. EPA 23 ff.; 38; 111.
[5] Cf. EPA 25 f.
[6] Cf. EPA ch. V.
[7] Cf. E. Tremblay, "Nature et définition de l'acte medical," *Laissez-les vivre* (Paris: Lethielleux, 1975) 333-336.
[8] Cf. EPA 16, f; 77-98; 136.
[9] Cf. EPA 82.
[10] Cf. EPA 136.
[11] Cf. EPA 15.
[12] *Ibid.*
[13] Cf. EPA 33 f.; 59; 149.
[14] Cf. EPA 33 f.; 122.

VIII

THE ACTORS: DOCTORS AND MAGISTRATES

Has the practice of abortion changed the image of medicine? **52.**
    The legalization and "medicalization" of abortion initiated a radical change in our conception of the doctor and medicine.[1]

    The doctor who takes advantage of the legalization of abortion might have the impression of serving his patient by aborting her. It is nevertheless permissible to wonder about the doctor's attitude:

—Is this doctor still unconditionally at the service of life in its beginnings? Is he not putting his art at the service of those who are stronger? Isn't he sacrificing the existence of the weakest to the interests of the strongest?[2]

—Doesn't the doctor risk exercising his art for the preferences of the state or dominant groups? Doesn't he become a mercenary careful, not to protect life and health, but to serve a patron other than the sick?[3]

—We know that today there are doctors who sterilize, abort (which is the equivalent to inflicting terrible tortures on the fetus to put it to death), or practice active euthanasia, sometimes presented as "assisted suicide." We are witnessing an essentially qualitative change in the doctor-patient relationship (Cf. 55).[4]

—Furthermore, studies recently published show that some doctors plan to associate themselves with power, to participate in it, and even to ensure "management of life by the state." Who will bear the expense of this medical technocracy? The so-called developed nations? The third world? The poor?[5]

    Whence the necessity for every doctor to make known without ambiguity his position regarding respect for life and his position vis-à-vis political power. Hence also the need for doctors who are unconditional servants of life to organize on an international level. To make oneself known is indispensable for being credible.

53. *Can one envisage a personality split among doctors?*

R. J. Lifton, one of the better contemporary specialists in Nazi medicine, quotes in this regard Dr. Miklos Nyiszli, prisoner doctor at Auschwitz: "The most dangerous of all criminals and assassins is the doctor assassin" (cf. 46, 75). And R. J. Lifton continues: "The doctor is dangerous, as we now see him, because of his ability to split himself in a way that invests his assassin Ego with special powers, all the while he continues to pride himself on his medical purity."[6]

54. *Should we not fear the interference of morality in the scientific domain?*

Scientific activity is typically human behavior; by that very fact, like all human behavior, it is subject to moral norms. Just like every other man, the savant is a morally responsible being. We must denounce the myth of the autonomy of science pushed all the way to scientific amorality. If we don't, we will reach a point at which either the savant will draw an argument from his knowledge and savoir-faire in order to impose himself on others, or he may well place himself in the pay of political leaders who will make good use of them. The government of men cannot revert to a medical technocracy.

55. *How can doctors be led to subordinate the interest of the individual to that of society?*

We can observe a growing tendency to politicize medical activity. What does politicize mean here? A doctor is one who knows the laws of the "order" and "progress" of human existence in its biological dimension. This is why some assert that the doctor must contribute to the emergence of the new man who will improve generic humanity, that is to say the species (cf. 69).

On the basis of such premises, the doctor is progressively led to put himself at the service of the body social (cf. 52); he is no longer at the service of individuals. These are evaluated according to their utility or their harmfulness in the body social, which alone matters. There would be categories (cf. 56) of human beings — defined, for example, according to racial, medical and economic, etc. criteria — who would pose a threat of degeneration for the whole of the species (cf. 32).

56. *Isn't the practice of abortion going to change the image of magistrates?*

Legislation and "medicalization" of abortion signal a radical change in our conception of magistrates and judges:

—Experience shows that, in countries where abortion has been liberalized, judges have practically no possibility of bringing about respect for the law (cf. 49).

—What is worse still is that most of the legislation liberalizing abortion transfers to the doctor the competence of a judge. We are in the present of a new case of alienation. The judge is removed from his original function: to make life respected before making property respected.

—It follows from that that judges henceforth will be better equipped to make property respected than to effect respect for the life of certain categories of human beings. They are even better equipped to protect the life of a criminal than that of an innocent person! If judges are "alienated," that is, deprived of their competence to effect respect for the unborn infant, they will also be powerless when it comes to insisting on respect for the elderly, the incurables, those who stand in the way, etc.

57. *How will the attitude of judges who fail to pursue their duty impact on political society?*

The attitude of judges who abstain from repressing abortion is always invoked to make an impression on legislators. The latter then are inclined to replace the judge in the evaluation of circumstances.

Besides, the legislator does not stop on such safe ground: he finally comes to request that the executive suggest that judges suspend their pursuits.

Thus legislation on abortion shows how real is the danger of confusion of powers (cf. 58).

58. *Would legislation liberalizing abortion threaten the separation of powers and by that fact the democratic quality of our societies?*

The vote for laws liberalizing abortion set in motion a process that renders very precarious the separation of powers — an essential criterion of a democratic society. In Western law, this separation receives a special clarification arising from the distinction between human rights and positive law.

The legislator must bring himself to elaborate just laws, that is to say, respectful of the inalienable rights of men. He expresses juridical norms, formulates rights and duties, stipulates penalties sanctioning violation of law. The legislator's activity, therefore, transpires on a general level that confers on law a transpersonal character. His role is not to apply the law.

Applying the law is the judge's role. It belongs to judicial power to evaluate the subjective responsibility of those who have been warned about objective infractions of the law. The judge will not deny the reality of the crime, but, in the determination of the penalty, he will take into account attenuating or aggravating circumstances.

The legislator who makes laws to serve the interests of particular persons, groups or lobbies gives proof of his partiality, injustice, arbitrariness, abuse of power. At the same time the judge who is content with a mechanical and blind application of the law also winds up being arbitrary and unjust.

Therefore it is clear what a risk to the separation of powers legislation about respect for life truly runs. Should the legislator make laws to serve the interests of a foreign power, he would be guilty of high treason. While the legislator exceeds his power by abusively broadening the sphere of his competence, the judge is reduced to executing more or less arbitrary determinations of the legislature. Is it necessary to say that this danger is exacerbated when the law comes directly from the executive's will? Law, and with it the magistrates, then risk becoming mere appendages of the administration.

[1] Cf. EPA ch. III.

[2] Cf. EPA 41.

[3] Cf. EPA 37 ff.; cf. DTL 165.

[4] Cf. EPA 39.

[5] Cf. EPA ch. XIV.

[6] See Robert Jay Lifton, *Les médecins nazis. Le meurtre médical et la psychologie du génocide* (Paris: Robert Laffont, 1989) 502.

IX

THE POLITICAL VIEWPOINT

How shall we define the political dimension of abortion? **59.**

The liberalization of abortion calls into question the "golden rule," that is, the principle that underlies all democracy: "Do not do unto others what you would not have them do to you" (cf. 114, 143). This prescription is but the negative formulation of the principle of the absolute respect we owe to others. Any violation of this principle weakens the very foundation of democracy: the original equality among men is the equality of all regarding the right to live. All other rights depend on that (cf. 1).

Nonetheless, isn't there any possibility of an exception to this rule? **60.**

One must take into account that when we consider abortion, we are talking about suppressing a human life. This point is no longer contested, even by the great majority of promoters of abortion (cf. 3). *The ultimate question, then, is to find out whether there exists a reason that permits putting an innocent person to death* (cf. 17, 68).

We might, for example, allege that one has the right to suppress those whose life, in our opinion, would not be worth living (cf. 71). At the beginning of the century, Karl Binding, a German lawyer, fabricated in this way a right "legitimizing" the suppression of those "whose life was not worth living": the sick, the elderly, the handicapped — the list could be made longer, since it was actually from this century.

Isn't it essential for a democratic society to promote the liberty of **61.** *individuals to the maximum?*

The desire to liberalize abortion is explained by a very restricted concept of freedom (cf. 37) that many of our contemporaries have (cf. 118-121). This concept is so extreme that it no longer allows for the idea of equality among men, nor, as a consequence, the idea of duty.

a) In this conception, freedom for each individual consists in doing whatever seems good to him, in behaving in whatever way pleases him. At each instant, individual conscience produces the moral norm that is convenient in such circumstances. Such a conception of freedom leads men to think that in their behavior there is no need to refer to a good they should seek or to an evil they should avoid. That is why, in his encyclical *Veritatis Splendor*, John Paul II reminds us that it is the truth which must direct freedom and not the opposite, and that truth is not "a creature of freedom."[1] No one can define good and evil as he pleases.

b) That is why in a society strongly marked by individualism everything, no matter what, becomes negotiable, from abortion to euthanasia going through all the forms of discrimination. No longer is there a search for good together; no longer is any effort made to aim at justice. *The very idea of the common good is emptied* of meaning: only individual good exists. Society no longer knows anything but compromise. We must exchange our viewpoints with fair play, in total tolerance (cf. 62) of what each one regards at the moment as good or bad.

In order to avoid at all costs the inconveniences of living together with other individuals, in order to avoid falling into anarchy, particular interests must be harmonized. All options are "equally respectable," but for reasons of utility or interest that does not prevent adhering to a purely "procedural" morality.[2] This is the triumph of committees for ethics, in which one proceeds stroke by stroke without reference to normative, universally binding, moral principles. Whence comes the appeal to the tyranny of the majority (cf. 42) and the tactic of dispensation (cf. 3). Particularly in this last case, they transfer the process of casuistry to law: just as this corrupts morality, so the tactic of dispensation perverts law. They reject at once any reference to general principles of law to accommodate the law to the pleasures and interests of those they wish to please.[3] This is but the triumphant return of sophistry.[4] What is forbidden here and now can be allowed tomorrow, for the only thing that matters at all times and places is to disturb people as little as possible and, of course, to be disturbed as little as possible.

c) From that point on there is no longer place for a morality binding on everyone and that underlies the very tissue of our human community. In effect, in such a conception of freedom, *everything is relativized.* The very idea of an *universal* Declaration of Human Rights is void of meaning. There are only individuals, and the violently emotional exaltation of freedom of each one guarantees a future of overexcited divisions among men.

d) Western democracies are fading away because, instead of relating to values, like truth, justice, solidarity, they are governed by a consensus reached through decisions that are purely procedural. National or international, political assemblies have become, so to speak, big committees on ethics in which the strongest try to impose a consensus according to their own interests.

e) Hence, it is impossible to create a more just and human society wherever, in order to achieve this end, one refuses to acknowledge that all men have the same fundamental rights.

f) In brief, this ultra-individualist conception of freedom turns against freedom, In such a conception, the political dimension of human existence is totally impugned and one sinks into anarchy. Anarchy is at once the absence of principles, and hence of legitimate authority, and therefore of government safeguarding the common good.

Doesn't tolerance mean that all opinions are respectable, including those   **62.**
of advocates of abortion and euthanasia?

a) Democratic societies that have emerged during the modern epoch all make reference to the universality of Human Rights. It is on this foundational reference that diverse positive prescriptions seeking to guarantee rights are engrafted. The right to life, to liberty, to property is the object of variable legal dispositions, but it is always these fundamental rights that are protected. It is the same for pluralism as for tolerance: it is always exercised in the framework of respect for the fundamental rights of man (cf. 42). In this sense, one understands what *civil tolerance* is: it is nothing else but the recognition and respect of persons (cf. 59). In this sense also, the modern state is civilly tolerant and pluralist.[5]

b) Those who violate, by legal means, the fundamental right to life of every human being defeat this civil tolerance and arrogate to themselves, as a consequence, the "right" to dispose of the existence of unborn infants and "useless" beings.

c) Whence comes the curious paradox of demolishing *civil tolerance* in the name of *doctrinal tolerance* or *doctrinal pluralism*. In effect, by reason of the latter, there is nothing but "procedural" ethics since all opinions are "equally respectable" (cf. 61). Hence, if the opinion that such and such a category of human beings isn't worthy of life triumphs, then the human beings listed under this rubric (by majority decision, of course) can be legally eliminated.

d) This conception of *doctrinal tolerance* and *doctrinal pluralism* thus signals the banishment of civil tolerance in any given society.

63. *Why does a state have a role to play regarding abortion?*

The quality of a state is measured first of all by the esteem in which it holds human life. When men enter political society, they expect that the state will protect, not only property and liberty, but above all life itself (cf. 42). The liberalization of abortion goes against this dynamic. Such liberalization means not only that protection of the law is refused some human beings (cf. 41, 43); it further entails the destruction of natural solidarity before it can even blossom. In the end, this process is the destroyer of the family and of the very tissue of society (cf. 6, 123).

Campaigns for the liberalization of abortion already had as their purpose — and this was stated by some — to destroy the child because he is the weakest link in the family chain. The principal and ultimate stake in the debates on bioethics pursued as a consequence of the study entrusted to professor Jean-François Mattei is the hastening of this process of destruction of the family.

Pioneer in the legalization of abortion, France risks besmirching its image even more on the international level by making the destruction of the family the priority of some kind of a republican messianism. This form of lay gallicanism cannot but wind up in the destruction of the social fabric, that is in hell itself.

64. *Doesn't the fact of taking the life of the innocent reveal a perversion of power?*

Totalitarian power has this characteristic in particular: it admits of no limit coming from God nor any control by the men over whom it is exercised. This power makes use of all the means at its disposal to assert and extend itself. Now, *power should be a service*: it is in the service of the common good and ordained to the protection of man, beginning with the weakest. All the great social movements that developed since the nineteenth century have contested the abuses of power committed by the strong against the weak.

The clearest sign indicating that an originally legitimate power is drifting toward totalitarianism is when it begins to take the lives of the innocent. Once this dynamic begins, power is debased into pure might and is deprived of all legitimacy. Such a power is abusive; it must be denounced and fought against; it makes active resistance a duty.

If the threat of totalitarianism were real, would it not be perceived by **65.** *everybody and would they not raise a general outcry?*

Contemporary history teaches us that totalitarianism is established sometimes by force, sometimes by ruse. In the latter case, its establishment is accomplished by strict adherence to the so-called "salami tactic": one conquers his adversary slice by slice; he would never give up if all were demanded at once. The "salami tactic" is thus close to the tactic of dispensation: they nibble away at the respect due to a principle by having the law multiply and make commonplace the cases in which positive law "justifies" whatever exception is made.

Evil begins whenever an iniquitous law is promulgated. It is consummated whenever such a law is invoked to massacre beings without defense. For the rest, at that moment the process can begin all over again, and new victims can be enrolled on the list of beings subject to massacre. Now, if some people are condemned for having obeyed evil laws, it is too often forgotten that others have been condemned for having intervened from above, that is, for having promulgated these evil laws and made the others executors of them.

Whence, when we arrive at asking the state to determine which innocent people can be eliminated, something authorized by law and for which a minister provides the means, then it is already too late to wonder whether we are still in a democracy.

[1] These themes are central to the enclyclical *Veritatis Splendor.* See in particular the whole of Ch. II, nos. 28-83, especially no. 35.

[2] See the discussions provoked by the work of John Rawls, *A Theory of Justice*, Oxford University Press, 1971.

[3] Cf. Pierre Cariou, *Pascal et la casuistique*, Paris: PUF, 1993.

[4] Cf. EPA 89-101.

[5] We have anallyzed this problem in *Droits de l'homme et technocratie* (Chambray: C.I.D., 1982) 28-32, and in *Démocratie et libération chrétienne* (Paris: Lethielleux, 1985) 70 f.

X

TOWARD ULTRA-NAZIISM

Would abortion be a modern form of discrimination? **66.**

History abounds with examples of discrimination (cf. 4). It also teaches that fighting against such discrimination and the privileges that accompanied it had been one of the powerful incentives toward democratic societies.

Now, to discriminate is always to invoke reasons for sending some human beings to their death or to slavery. Sometimes to discriminate is to increase an objective weakness twofold by adding a legal weakness.

The Nazi regime discriminated against the Jews, gypsies and the "un-human" (cf. 60). At Nuremberg that was called a "crime against humanity"; since then the memory of men has been relieved of such bothersome recollections.[1]

Other regimes discriminated against those who disagreed or opposed them by sending them, for example, to psychiatric asylums. And now they discriminate against, not only infants and adults who are deformed or handicapped (cf. 67), but also the poor (cf. 80-93).

Liberalization of abortion legalized a new kind of discrimination which can make victims, with impunity, those who find themselves in a state of extreme weakness and dependence.

Isn't the ideology that inspires the promoters of abortion entirely **67.**
different from that of the Nazis?

There are at the same time some different expressions but a profound commonality of inspiration. Explicit justifications are presented in different packaging, but the practices to which they lead are ultimately the same (cf. 142). Whether one speaks of Jew, gypsy, the handicapped, the unborn infant, the undesired infant, or the incurable adult, once it comes to eliminating them, the motives invoked may differ but the horror is the same. What difference does it make if the ideologies vary but the practices are the same?

68. *Still must we not concede that even if the practices are the same the ideologies themselves are different?*

The ideological reasons forged in order to "legitimize" Naziism and abortion do not resort to the same formulation, but they have this in common that they "legitimize" *absolutely arbitrary discrimination* among human beings.

Whence the points common to the ideologues of genocide and the promoters of abortion: in both cases the victim is not recognized as a human being; in both cases the victim is innocent (cf. 60, 64).

And to that we must add the fact that, if we are to believe the statistics of WHO (cf. 2), the annual victims of abortions are incomparably more numerous that the victims of Nazi genocide.

69. *What link is there between the ideologues of discrimination and the medical engineers?*

a) The ideologues of discrimination concoct some pseudo-moral reasons to explain to the complacent medical engineers that they are justified in eliminating those beings who do not fit the norms imposed by the ideology.

These ideologues make sure that the biomedical engineers are sufficiently "grounded" to perform the rigid selections "for the good" of certain individuals, of such and such a race, of society of the species — it depends!

Thus, having striven so hard to put a stop to segregation based on "social classes," the men of our century now hurry to establish a new segregation based on "genetic classes."

b) The ideologues of discrimination provide a pseudo-legitimation to multiple *abuses of power.* Contemptible indeed is the abuse of economic, political and judicial power. More contemptible still is the abuse of medical power. But the most contemptible of all is the abuse of intellectual power, for it wounds man in his very intelligence in which he is most like God (cf. 140).

The technocrats of the new world order are accustomed to these refined forms of the abuse of power.

70. *Aren't we finding here again criteria invoked for the profit of society that are analogous to those invoked for the profit of couples?*

The arguments invoked by female partisans and other promoters of abortion are based on self-interest, utility, the right to pleasure without risk. They must have total effectiveness when it comes to avoiding this "evil" called procreation — the eventual consequence of this "good" called pleasure (cf. 122). Thus the stronger may believe that their convenience gives them the right to "legitimize" abortion.

a) The interests of human society are defined by the strongest, concretely by those who are successful and/or impose their will on others. Those who are not successful are an obstacle to the happiness of those who are. They threaten even their security. Consequently, the rich believe that their security is the basis of their right and are thus justified in defending themselves against the threats posed by the poor who, solely by their numerical mass, constitute a danger for them (cf. 137). Their proliferation must be contained by every possible means insofar as they are insolvent in the world market (cf. 97, 99).

b) This line of argumentation is analogous to that developed, if we dare say it, for the benefit of society (cf. 69). It has been verified since 1926 in the USSR, where abortion has been legalized so that the population could be totally subjected to the planning imperatives imposed by the state. The USSR was thus the first country to legalize abortion for reasons of state.

71. *Does not the refusal to accept all risk lead precipitously and ruthlessly down the spiral of pure effectiveness?*

Risk is intolerable both for the partisans of sexual freedom as well as society. That is why, beginning with contraception, the logic behind effectiveness leads through abortion, then eugenics (cf. 30), to end in euthanasia (cf.31).

A common idea underlies these different practices: when they say that a human life does not fit certain "norms of quality" and that it is not worth living, this life — they conclude — may be suppressed by the most effective means available.

72. *Can we really speak of abortions as "imprescriptible crimes against humanity"?*

After the second World War, once the magnitude of Nazis atrocities became better known, the "crimes against humanity"[2] were denounced. Besides the war crimes and the crimes against peace, it was above all this chief accusation that was principally pursued at the Nuremburg trial.

These crimes include murder, mass extermination, genocide, torture, arbitrary arrest, etc. Ever since the Convention was adopted on November 26, 1968, by the general assembly of the United Nations, these crimes against humanity have been considered *imprescriptible,* that is, they can never be ordered. They are thus precisely because they must always be condemned in the name of a law inscribed on the heart of man and anterior to all positive legislation. On the contrary, positive legislation is subject to the sanction of the law inscribed in the heart of man.

What was emphasized at Nuremburg is that the Nazi crimes could not be prescribed *because* they were committed in the name of evil laws. Yes, they were evil laws because they did not respect the inalienable rights of every human being.

The Universal Declaration of Human Rights of 1948 would draw its teaching both from this war and trial. It would make more explicit, it would proclaim the ultimate reasons why we had to — and must always — fight against Naziism, condemn its crimes and prevent its resurgence.

The liberalization of abortion calls into question again the very principles upon which was based the condemnation of Naziism.

73. *Is it possible to forget the evident lessons arising from the Nazi experience?*

Men have a prodigious capacity for hiding the past — and the present — even if they have suffered in their own flesh. They practice a sort of *damnatio memoriae*: memory is condemned, for the past is perceived as dangerous, since knowledge of it allows them to judge the present (cf. 76 f.).

Thus we make it difficult for ourselves to take into account that it was under the pretext of obedience to the laws of the Third Reich and to the orders of superiors that Nazi doctors and other torturers executed innocent masses. And we further fail to take into account that we were saved from Naziism *precisely because the resistance disobeyed the laws because they were evil*. And lets us face the fact that, by a macabre return of history, some who survived that Nazi horror thanks to the resistance are today endeavoring to restore evil laws entirely similar to those the liberators refused to obey in order to save them. . .

Now, just as these facts of contemporary history have been hidden, it is clear that also hidden is the fact that history can repeat itself or, if you prefer, can be prolonged. And just as clearly, it is in the name of laws, no longer imposed by tyrants, but voted in by parliaments that the innocent are executed.

74. *Does fidelity to the memory of the victims suffice to vaccinate us against a new barbarism?*

a) Among those who endeavor to have approved the unjust laws by which people without defense are executed some are numbered who reproach — justly — the Nazi torturers for having obeyed criminal laws.

Yesterday, that is at Nuremburg, the accused retreated behind unjust laws in the attempt to excuse their crimes; today one asks the legislator to grant similar crimes the protection of the law.

b) At least one should not invoke the sacrifice of these innocent people of yesterday to consider himself authorized to introduced, today, the principle of new legal discrimination among human beings. The sacrifice of the martyrs of old totalitarian regimes is a sacred thing. No one can retreat behind the memory of these deaths to pretend himself immunized against the present totalitarian trends.

c) One would wish that none of those who suffered from Nazi barbarism would reject, either in theory or in practice, the always present arguments which were invoked in their favor and against their torturers by those who gave testimony, that all men without distinction have the same dignity, the same right to life and liberty.

How do we explain these inconsistencies that lead to legalize today **75.**
practices that yesterday were condemned as illegitimate?

The inconsistency which we have just analyzed (cf. 73) is dramatic, for it reveals that in certain quarters people haven't perceived the profound malice of Naziism. That is why the door is wide open to ultra-Naziism. By that we mean a Naziism brought to its supreme stage, made global and inscribed in practices, laws, institutions and even ethics.[3]

a) People haven't understood that this malice does not reside first of all in the *regime* which Naziism characterizes but deep in the nature of the latter. They haven't seen that the essence of Naziism is its totalitarian nature, that is to say its desire to *destroy the Ego*, both physically as well as psychologically. Naziism is haunted by the desire to inflict death (cf. 142).

b) Despite the loud denials of those who are animated by currents which, after legalizing abortion, are now endeavoring to legalize euthanasia (cf. 30-32), these currents are *objectively* inscribed with the Nazi tradition, and while drinking in its perversion, they go well beyond it. In effect, to inflict death is not just a "right" that society may exercise on the life it regards unworthy of living [4](cf. 60); it is also a "duty" whose execution the same society must guarantee for those who desire to "die with dignity" because their life is not worth living (cf. 30).

43

Added to the consideration of the right of society to inflict death on beings whose life isn't worth living, typical of Naziism (cf. 60), is a consideration typical of liberalism: the right of the individual to "die with dignity."

c) But in these two scenarios, and beyond the ideological travesties, the act of inflicting death is covered by law and its execution is entrusted to medical personnel. In brief, the law now legitimizes medical murder (cf. 46, 53).

d) For the same reasons, once a state grants parents the "right" to kill their children, it quickly finishes by granting children the "right" to kill their parents (cf. 30-32, 52).

Thus, in these different cases, the "law" is called upon to legitimize the "medicalization" of murder (cf. 46, 53).

e) This totalitarian alliance between the lie and violence was implacably denounced by Andre Frossard: "The liar knows that he lies, the criminal hides or denies his crime, and the political systems that are the most diabolically injurious to the human species believe themselves constrained to give a decor of justice to their ignominies, and to feign a right each time it violates it."[5]

76. *Recalling the past can be disturbing for some. But for those who today perfect, manufacture and distribute abortifacients, is it not as disturbing to emphasize the effectiveness of their products?*

a) It is well known that men have a great facility for giving apparently coherent "justifications" that inspire their conduct, all the while hesitating to look squarely in the face the deep motivations that animate them. This type of behavior is well known among psychologists who speak about "rationalizing" conduct. More or less voluntarily, men can hide from themselves or from others the true motives that prompt their behavior.

b) This is what happens sometimes among certain propagators of chemical abortion. As circumstances allow, they do not insist too much on the essentially abortive power of their preparations (cf. 96). On the other hand, they emphasize the effectiveness — real or supposed — in cases of breast cancer , endometrial cancer, brain cancer, Alzheimer's disease, depression, etc. [6]

c) One observes: this "rationalization" recalls the *damnatio memoriae*, the condemnation of memory (cf. 73). Here, one hides an embarrassing past; there one hides bothersome actual motives. These two processes often intertwine in order to reinforce the cover-up effect.

Despite all, isn't it very unlikely that those who have perfected and   **77.**
commercialized effective methods of chemical abortion are
totally insensitive to the lessons of the past?

The phenomenon of *damnatio memoriae,* condemnation of memory, is characteristic of all the groups who have a bad conscience (cf. 73, 76).

a) They erase the past first of all because they are ashamed of it. Some old imperial powers still restrict their archives relative to their conquests. Some colonies, independent for a long time, have destroyed almost all of the documents relating to slavery.

But they erase the past also because they are afraid to risk illuminating the present and thus being able to judge it. This fear is particularly frequent among societies with a strong totalitarian design. Mao Tse-tung purged the history of Chinese culture because the Chinese of communist China would have already found there ample material for demystifying the ideology of the Great Leader. Knowledge of the past and its remembrance were rejected because they would have brought them to an *alarming realization.* The reactivation of memory, by recalling history, is thus perceived as out of place, *impertinent* even, because it can brutally unmask the deceitful certitudes of a bad conscience.

b) In the case with which we are concerned, this reactivation could, for example, lead to asking whether a new genocide is not about to unfold. This genocide would no longer have as victims those envisaged by historical Naziism; today the immense multitude of poor people above all would be targeted. An observer as perspicacious as concerned, Dr. Baulieu, affirms that "in accord with the World Health Organization, the Hoechst Company decided that in the countries of the Third World, which represent the real big markets, the pill [RU 486] would be sold at a much lower price or given away gratis."[7]

c) In the case of the Hoechst laboratory which, together with Roussel-Uclaf, produced the RU 486 pill (cf. 95 f.), fear of bringing up the past has been cleverly analyzed by the same Dr. Baulieu. In an interview granted to the Italian review *L'Espresso,* he noted that: "It was precisely the directors of the American affiliate of Hoechst that poisoned the opinion of the German mother company. Hilger, its president, even as a Bavarian Catholic never had anything against the pill. But today he is afraid. And his fears are nourished by certain phantoms of the past. The Hoechst firm was founded after the war from the dismantlement of the I. G. Farben Co., the industrial giant that, among others, produced the gas for the Nazi extermination camps. Hilger is in terror of the idea that anti-abortion groups will let loose a campaign accusing Hoechst of continuing to kill as in the Hitler days"[8] (cf. 46).

If we understand this "terror" well, we understand less, on the other hand, the block that limits the perception of the firm's president.

78. *Isn't it shocking to suggest a parallel between the Nazi torturers and the abortionists of today?*

People often imagine that the Nazi type was a ferocious and bloodthirsty individual. This type of Nazi most certainly existed, ignoble individuals rivaled one another in refining ways of inflicting humiliation, torture and death.

But generally speaking, the classical Nazi was not a cruel brute. In the main, the Nazis were people apparently without history, like the majority of people today. They had simply entered the "system" tranquilly. With one concession after another, and cowardly act after cowardly act (cf. 65), and with self-interest they became zealous functionaries of the regime. By executing their orders, they did their duty—so they believed.[9]

The greater peril that the liberalization of abortion today has hanging over our societies, is not to be looked for first of all in the actions of individuals notoriously cynical and ruthless. It is found in the generalized lack of courage in face of "commonplace evil."[10]

[1] Cf. DTL 265.

[2] See Maurice Torelli, *Le médecin et les droits de l'homme* (Paris: Berger-Levrault, 1983) 236-238.

[3] See EPA, 179-187; DTL 265-268.

[4] See EPA 14, 132; DTL 127 f.; Cf. R. J. Lifton, *Les médecins nazis* (cited at question 53) 64 f.

[5] Cf. André Frossard, *Défense du Pape* (Paris: Fayard, 1993) 48.

[6] See the dossier of Carlo Galluci on "La pillola maldetta," *L'Espresso* (Rome, Oct. 20, 1991) 156-165, esp. 163.

[7] See *ibid*. 163.

[8] See *ibid*. 161. See also the discussion between Edouard Sakiz and Dr. J. Y. Nau in *Le Monde* of April 27, 1993. In this discussion they report the fear that the boycott of RU 486 inspired in the USA as well as Hilger's attitude. On the role of I. G. Farben under the Nazi regime, see R. J. Lifton, *Les médecins nazis* (cited at question 53); see also the index p. 602.

[9] Cf. DTL 267.

[10] Cf. DTL 266-268.

XI

THE DEMOGRAHPIC ASPECTS

What can one actually say about world population?   **79.**
    a) In December of 1993, the world population was estimated at 5,543,000,000 inhabitants.[1]

    b) On the world scale, "growth has slowed: it was already but 1.7% in 1990 where as it had been 2.1% a year earlier; and the absolute number is going to decrease a little after the year 2000, *having taken into account the drop in fertility already recorded in numerous developing countries.*"[2]

    c) The phenomenon of spectacular growth of population "occurred with an accelerated rhythm in countries of the South in the 20th century. This rhythm, however, has begun to drop, because world fertility began to diminish with a swiftness that is not negligible in the countries of the Third World: 6.1 infants a woman in 1962, around 3.8 infants a woman in 1990."[3] Practically all over, the synthesized indices of fertility (cf. 85) have dropped.

At least a fifth of humanity lives in a situation of absolute poverty, in   **80.**
subhuman conditions, unworthy of man. For the sake of these
people and their families, would it not be better to prevent them
from having children?
    a) The Malthusians assert that there is a disparity between the geometric progression of the population and the arithmetic increase of food resources. The Neomalthusians combine this thesis with that of the right to individual sexual pleasure without risk of procreation. The Neomalthusian theses — proposing contraception, sterilization, abortion, etc. as the new "rights of man" — are very frequently used as a deception making the Malthusian motive of those who consider strict control of the population a "duty" as urgent as it is imperative (cf. 88).

    These intertwined theses are spread throughout the entire world by those who see their own interests served thereby.[4]

b) Poverty is not a fatality, nor is hunger. *Surplus food*, for example, has never been so important. It is the same for *life expectancy* at birth, which has never been very high anywhere in the world. But there are serious problems of distribution, not only in what concerns food resources. but also, for example, in agricultural know-how, health, hygiene, the natural regulation of birth, etc. — not counting corruption.[5] What the poor expect is that they be given aid to get out of their misery, not that they be left to stagnate after having been "offered" abortion and sterilization.

c) Mass sterilization of the poor, as it is actually being practiced, is going to have terrible consequences.[6] When they get old they will still be as poor, but they won't have any children to count on. They will be abandoned, and the violence done to them by society will accelerate their death, as it has already left to die the street urchins no one would take care of.

d) Presented today in a new wrapping, Malthus' theses are more than ever an instrument for dreaming on the part of all those reactionaries opposed to every social reform. The Malthusians of today are indoctrinating international opinion by having it swallow the idea that poverty doesn't find its cause in social injustice, or in economic failure, or in political incompetence, or in ideological aberrations. According to them, poverty has its source in the dizzying proliferation of poor people themselves. It follows that, to the degree that this thesis, though false, is inculcated and accepted as blinding "evidence," true appeals for justice and development may be ignored and the exploitation of the poor can be pursued without scruples.

e) Malthus has thus become today the standard bearer for all those who are an obstacle to social justice — among men and among nations — to universal fraternity, equality, freedom for all, to respect for the weak, the poorest, the handicapped, the ailing, etc. For the Malthusians of today, the poor, the weak, the Blacks, the Indians, etc. are despicable; equality of all men, the right of all to freedom, access of all to material, intellectual and spiritual goods — all these are so many inadmissible objectives that must be fought against. To take care of the weak, to promote equal dignity for all men upsets, according to them, the equilibrium willed by nature, which selects the fittest and eliminates the weakest.

In sum, Malthusian ideas inspire the contemporary version of morality — naturalist and Nietzschean — of the "lords." In this sense, these ideas are totally incompatible with Christianity.

Won't it contribute to the happiness of the poor to have access to   **81.**
   sterilization and abortion made easier?

The rich seem to have at their disposal a mysterious machine called a *eudaemometer*, an apparatus that enables them to measure happiness: their appreciation is in fact based upon statistics relating to revenue.[7] With that as their starting point, the rich estimate that the life of the poor has no sense because they have little revenue; it's necessary then, they say, to prevent the poor from having children (cf. 10). The life of the poor would be worth the trouble if they had access to pleasure and to the wealth that opens the way to it. And so abortion and sterilization are recommended, thus making them believe they will be less poor and, above all, have access to pleasure.

Moreover, it is the same for individuals as for nations: there is no worse humiliation for a nation than massive sterilization of its citizens. This mutilation is, alas, frequently accompanied by a lie, since one "offers," by way of "aid to poor countries," what in the city is sometimes imposed as a punishment on those condemned for sexual crimes.

Isn't a terrible threat hanging over humanity: the "demographic   **82.**
   explosion" of the Third-World?

This notion goes back to the Malthusian theories. According to Malthus (1766-1834), population increases in a *geometric* progression and the food resources in an arithmetic one (cf. 80). This theory has resurfaced today in a barely modified form: "People are poor because they are too numerous." This assertion is broadcast by the media which try hard to impose as blinding evidence that "to be numerous is to be poor."

But we must not say that people are poor because they are too numerous but that *they are too numerous because they are poor* (cf. 83). To restrain births energetically in order to put an end to poverty is to approach the problem in the reverse.

Population excess is always measured *in relationship* to a precise, concrete and variable situation. Poverty is always evaluated according to man's capacity to face his environment: a nation is poor because it isn't able to feed it's population. (cf. 92). In this sense, poverty is the cause of overpopulation and not the reverse; overpopulation is always relative to a given situation.[8] Now this situation can be *changed by man's intervention on the condition that he has both the moral and political desire to do so.* There are cases in which people are so materially, intellectually and morally under-equipped that they have no possibility of being properly educated and therefore are, in fact, in this situation too numerous.. But that is the point: man can change these situations by organization, teaching and by supplying equipment (cf. 137).[9]

That doesn't mean that the demographic phenomena should not be taken into account; here there is decline, there growth.[10] Public authority must, then, take care of this problem. But here as elsewhere one must *respect the principle of subsidiarity*, the basis of all democracy.[11] The intervention of public authorities must be accomplished always with respect to the fundamental rights of man. They may not use just any means at any price.

83. *Some go so far as to speak of a "demographic bomb" all ready to explode.*

In the eyes of the ideologues of demographic security, to be numerous is to be poor. But the bomb of the 3rd millenium is the poverty of the Third World, not the poor. Here as elsewhere, one must not err in diagnosing the problem or in confusing the effect with ts cause (cf. 82, 137, 141).

a) The causes of poverty cannot be resolved by sterilizing the poor (cf. 82, 107) — no more than sickness can be remedied by euthanizing the sick (cf. 30 f.). In order to remedy the causes of poverty, *it is most urgent that all children receive an education* that allows them, by the time they are adults, to meet their needs, and we must help them get it (cf. 82).

b) It would be very difficult to find historical examples of a development that followed upon a drop in the birth rate.

c) In Brazil, from 1960 to 1990, the general rate of fertility, that is to say, the annual number of births relative to the number of women of childbearing age, went from 6.3 to 3.13, while the rate of demographic growth went from 2.89% to 1.8%. Can one say that during this period poverty decreased as much?

84. *Does this fear of population growth in the Third World involve certain countries in particular?*

a) The *Report of the National Security Council*, also called the *Kissinger Report* (cf. 100-102) explains that developing countries must be the first targeted by the anti-birth campaigns:

Emphasis must be placed primarily on the developing countries that are the biggest and that grow more rapidly and where the disequilibrium between the increasing number [of inhabitants] and the development potential entails the most serious risks of instability, unrest and international tensions. These countries are: India, Bangladesh, Pakistan, Nigeria, Mexico, Indonesia, Brazil, The Philippines, Thailand, Egypt, Turkey, Ethiopia and Colombia.[12]

b) As important as it is, this report is not unique of its kind, numerous other documents confirm that constant determination shown by the North American authorities.[13]

How is the demographic situation in Europe? 85.

In order to insure that population reproduces itself in the "developed" countries, the rate of fertility must be 2.1 children per woman. This index is calculated for one determined year by adding the quotients of fertility by age. This should be explained: they report the number of children born during a determined year to the number of women aged 15 to 49 on January 1st of the year in question and these partial quotients are added.

For example, for a given region, they report the number of children born in 1990 to the number of women 15 years old on January 1, 1990. Thus a partial quotient is obtained, called also quotient of fertility by age or rate of partial fertility. One does the same calculation for infants born in 1990 but to women 16 years old on January 1, 1990, and on up to 49 years old. Then these quotients for the same year are all added up to obtain the *synthesized fertility index* for the year.[14]

Almost everywhere in Europe, this fertility index is *clearly below the level necessary for population replacement*.[15] For the *European community*, the data published in 1993 by *Eurostat* reports a fertility index that was 2.61 in 1960 and dropped to 1.51 in 1991. Ireland alone, with an index of 2.10 is assured of reproducing itself. Be the judge: always according to *Eurostat*, the last fertility index available gives 1.82 for the United Kingdom, 1.62 for Belgium, 1.33 for Germany, 1.33 for Spain, 1.26 for Italy.[16] For France, the same *Eurostat* (1993) gives 1.78, but a recent study by Guy Herzlich in *Le Monde* of Feb. 10, 1994, reports 1.65 for the year 1993.

The drop is even more spectacular in the countries of *Eastern Europe*: "The number of children per woman has literally tumbled in eastern Germany: from nearly 1.6 in mid-1990 to .83 in 1992. But Russia has fallen in two years from 1.9 to 1.56. . . . Catholic Poland returned to 1.95 children per woman as has Slovakia. . . . In Russia since the end of 1991, the total number of deaths exceeded that of births."[17] Just in the years 1965-1970 the synthesized fertility index in Europe had been almost everywhere above 2.1. By way of comparison, let us indicate that this index, which declined almost on all the continents since 1965 (cf. 79), was estimated at 3.3 for the whole world and at 3.7 for the Third World.[18]

86. *How has Europe come to such a demographic collapse?*

The causes of this demographic implosion are obviously complex. In any case, there is one that merits emphasis. In order to make contraception, sterilization and abortion acceptable in the Third World, Europe had itself to "give the example." The message Europe addressed to the poor countries would not have been credible if it hadn't itself begun to adopt and legalize these practices. Since 1973 the agronome René Dumont wrote: "*Authoritarian* measures for limiting birth. . . are going to become more and more necessary, but they will not be acceptable *unless they begin in the rich countries* and through education of the others.[19]

European example did bring about its effect of imitation in the Third World, but in addition it had a *boomerang effect* in Europe. This is a new version of the story of the trick backfiring: Europe had been and continues to be the first victim of the "anti-life" practices it wanted to export to the Third World to insure its keeping control.

87. Doesn't the United States also experience a demographic collapse comparable to that of Europe?

Despite appearances, from the demographic viewpoint, the situation in the United States is different from that in Europe. First of all, its synthesized fertility index (cf. 85) of 2.0 is markedly above that of the European community where it is only 1.51 (cf. 85). Moreover it is well known that this fertility differs from ethnic group to ethnic group. For example, it is much higher among the Blacks and those of Latin-American origin than among the WASPs, that is to say, among the "White, Anglo-Saxon Protestants." We should note also that the pyramid of age is more balanced and the proportion of young people higher than in Europe.[20]

We should also report that the pro-life movements are much more active and better organized in the USA than in Europe. Their influence on the media is very important; their voices carry weight during elections; they have demonstrated many times the formidable use one can make of the boycott aimed at pharmaceutical firms (cf. 39). Recent presidents, like Reagan and Bush, have had to come to terms with them.

The *diversity* of demographic questions, depending on whether we speak of the Third World or Europe, finds its reflection in the *ambiguity* of relationships between Europe and the United States.

a) The United States and the Anglo-Saxon world in general have been pioneers in the area of contraception, sterilization and abortion. The main Malthusian and Neomalthusian theses continue to be widely spread from centers based in the USA or England. These countries have shared with Europe their obsession with "demographic security" regarding the Third World whose expansion they fear very much.

This communal interest leads Europe and the USA to join forces in order to restrict the demographic pressure of the Third World, and they don't hesitate to control international institutions to attain their end. They even seek in the new antagonism between the North and the South the cohesive cement which the previous East-West antagonism no longer assures them.

b) Nevertheless, beyond this community of interests, it appears more and more clear that the United States, obsessed with its security, wishes to *prevent the emergence of a new rival,* whoever it might be.[21]

The Third World in general is, in the end, a potential rival whose emergence must be controlled (cf. 84). Let us mention rapidly two examples:

—first of all China: it "benefits" from an "aid" to demographic control the breadth and effectiveness of which have recently been denounced (cf. 106, 125);

—then Mexico: a country developing in step with the city, it must be watched more closely; and it is since being integrated into a "free market" regrouping the states of North America.

Of different concern, however, is the maintainance of European power with the organization of the European Union.

c) One can wonder if Europe is not in the process of itself destroying its ability to intervene in favor of the development of the Third World. By consenting to its demographic decline, Europe gives more elbow room to the United States. For all that, it could offer poor countries the alternative solution of partnership — if it had not let itself get caught in a trap.

d) It follows, therefore, that, in looking at things this way, the United States has all the reason in the world to rejoice over the demographic collapse of Europe. For the same reasons, it has grounds for being satisfied with Europe's *aging*,[22] insofar as this will inevitably entail social difficulties from the moment that the policies about social security, sickness, disability and retirement are called into question — in fact, this has already widely begun!

Under the influence of opinion makers (perhaps under pay), the paralyzed European community, hurriedly introduced the Neomalthusian ideology of the right to pleasure, originally an Anglo-Saxon idea. At the same time it was in the interest of the United States that Europe, yielding to *Malthusian* behavior, *strictly contain* (cf. 93, 96) *the growth of its own population* (cf. 80). The United States must, then, be laughing up its sleeve to see the haste with which the Europeans interiorized the very theses it spread everywhere! We never had such a good example of ideological colonization. . . .

e) It's about time that Europe and the Third World recalled the aphorism attributed to Disraeli: "The British Empire has no permanent enemies, nor permanent friends. It has only permanent interests."

89. *Since the demographic situation of Europe is so grave, why are so few politicians concerned about it?*

The lack of attention shown by most European politicians to these demographic problems is really staggering. There are different reasons for that. First of all, most politicians perceive the problems connected with respect for life, *not in function of the common good but in function of their electorate.* If concern for the common good prevailed among them, the long term would be favored and the demographic problems would receive the proper attention they deserve. But politicians are generally more sensitive to the short and medium term. They care more about their own particular good, their re-election, then pleasing the electorate whom they must seduce in view of the next election.

Even Christian politicians who should have specific reasons to be concerned about these questions, often give proof of softness in these matters (cf. 116). The national and European parliaments have given a thousand examples of this. In particular, it is perfectly scandalous that Christian politicians have affixed their signatures to the laws regulating abortion.

Finally, we must never lose sight of the fact that *cultivated ignorance* is the superior form of voluntary servitude, although we must acknowledge that it finds formidable rivals in bad faith, corruption and lack of courage.[23]

How is the problem of abortion presented in a country like Japan   ***90.***
   where it has become commonplace?

Abortion is in effect practiced currently in Japan, and they estimate that there are a half a million a year. We must remark, however, that this frequency of abortion does not achieve a sense of guilt among those who have recourse to it. There are even cemeteries for unborn infants in which figurines represent the little victims of abortion.[24]

Japan, where few women work, is nevertheless going to pose a grave problem in regards to demography. The fertility index is 1.5,[25] and the aging of the population is accentuated.

Until now, Japan has prevented or skirted its demographic decline by establishing some of its industries in foreign countries. But the Japanese directors are realizing that the expansion of Japan risks being hypothetical by reason of the foreseeable difficulties due to the demographic dynamic.

That is why Japan has recently taken strict measures to prevent women from using contraception.

It is also the reason why Tokyo is trying to bring back to Japan emigrants and children of Japanese emigrants. This reverse migration has the objective of contributing to the resolution of the problem of lack of manpower in the Empire of the Rising Sun.

Has anyone an idea of the consequences of the collapse of fertility   ***91.***
   in the developed countries?

These consequences are many and varied and are foreseeable now. In a general way, a demographic imbalance between North and South cannot be seen as reassuring for the future of human society. The demographic collapse of the North would certainly entail a general weakening of the vitality of all of humanity.

Two consequences deserve, however, to be set in relief, for they concern the future of Europe and in particular of Western Europe:

a) The first is that the demographic collapse of Europe is going to reinforce the non-Europeans in their *migratory tendencies.* This is particularly true regarding the relationship between Europe and the Maghreb in North Africa. While in Europe the work force is decreasing, the population of the Maghreb, younger and more fertile, will bring an ever greater pressure on Europe, particularly Latin Europe. This population will be either underemployed in its own countries or employed via the European circuits of production. In both cases the problems risk being all the more delicate to manage as the experience of the recent past shows that Europe is not anxious to favor the integration of the Maghreb workers already established in its territory.[26]

b) The second consequence is by far the more serious; it is also the least easily perceived by the public at large. This consequence, as Pierre Chaunu has often insisted, is the *exhausting* of the tradition of culture and science.[27] In effect, in the final analysis, man is the sole, unique bearer of culture and knowledge. Culture, science, morals, religions are not transmitted except through the intervention of men who endlessly enrich them. *Humanity's memory* is a living memory, that is, creative and inventive. Written documents, the various "monuments" are dead realities if no one is there to interrogate them, dialogue with them and go beyond them (cf. 142). The major risk that Europe runs is, lacking manpower, culture will languish. Absent the numerous exchanges that a large and dense population stimulates, culture and science run a double mortal risk: repetitious stagnation, first of all, then finally shipwreck.

In the end, if Europe goes down, demographically speaking, its shipwreck will petrify the Third World in under-development and/or place it under the discretionary tutelage of the United States.

92. *Hasn't mankind, by its very mass, become a nuisance for the environment?*

It is certainly clear that man has a fantastic ability to destroy the environment.

a) If all men consumed as much and as anarchically as the inhabitants of rich countries, the planet would be burned up.

b) The setting on fire of the oil wells in the Gulf region proved that this destructive ability can go all the way to madness.[28] At the same time, the devastation of the Amazon is no less worrisome.

c) Disastrous effects, even if on a lesser scale, are produced wherever natural resources are exploited using archaic and ineffective methods that are damaging to the environment.

On the other hand,

a) The progress of agronomy, for example, happily shows that man has also an astonishing capacity for managing the environment and natural resources well. Even the Food and Agriculture Organization admitted that the problem of feeding mankind is less a technical problem that a political and therefore moral problem (cf. 82, 128).

b) Moreover, it is education and enrichment of the population that permit regulation of birth and not the inverse.

c) Finally, to respect the ecosystem is first of all to respect the heart of the environment, and that is the human being. How can one respect an elephant or a baby seal if one does not even respect the flesh of one's flesh?

What so often happens is that, drawn by the unbridled lure of gain, some people destroy the natural equilibrium, then, with a rare cynicism they declare that there are too many people on the planet earth and that this "overpopulation" pollutes the ecosystem (cf. 137): They damage the Amazon region and then say that there are too many people in Brazil.[29]

[1] According to the review *Population Today* (Washington: Population Reference Bureau, Dec. 1993) 9.

[2] Guy Herzlich, "Le couple population-développement," *Le Monde*, Dec. 14, 1993. Our emphasis.

[3] Gerard-François Dumont, "Révolutions démographiques," *Le Spectacle du monde* no. 361 (April 1992) 80 f.

[4] Cf. DTL 146.

[5] Cf. Francis Gendreau (ed.), *Les spectres de Malthus* (Paris: Etudes et Documentation Internationales, 1991); see, for example, the Chapter devoted to Bangladesh 173-178. See also the work edited by Sylvie Brunel, *Tiers-Monde* cited in question 82.

[6] Cf. DTL 157 ff.

[7] Sharon L. Camp did not hesitate to publish a leaflet exposing *The Human Suffering Index*; this leaflet was published in Washington by the Population Crisis Committee, 1987.

[8] Cf. EPA, ch. XIV.

[9] On the problems considered in this section see EPA as well as DTL. See also Sylvie Brunet *Tiers-Monde, Controverses et Realités* (Paris: Ed. Economica, 1987). Cf. in particular the article, "La croissance démographique, frein. . . ou moteur du développement?" by Jean-Claude Chesnais with Alain Destexhe, Claude Albagi et Alain Guilloux, 119-177.

[10] See the remarkable dossier devoted to demography by the review *Défense nationale*, April 1993, 19-75. This dossier benefitted from the collaboration of Gerard-Fran-

çois Dumont, "La population au XXe siècle," (19-35); Id., "Démographie et géopolitique," (37-54); Yves Montenay, "Les politiques de natalité dans le tiers-monde" (55-65); Jean-Didier Lecaillon, "Les démographes se trompent-ils?" (67-74). On the demographic phenomena one will want to refer to the work of Gerard-François Dumont cited in question 85. Beside this reference work, we should also mention that of Jacques Veron, *Arithmétique de l'homme* (Paris: Seuil, 1993).

[11] According to the principle of subsidiarity, the public authorities must help individuals and intermediary entities, such as the family, to take the intiative that belongs to them and not substitute for them. About subsidiarity, see our work *Initiation à l'Enseignement social de l'Eglise* (Paris: Ed. de l'Emmanuel, 1992).

[12] The document NSSM 200, known under the title *Report of the National Security Council* or the *Kissinger Report*, carries the title, *Implications of Worldwide Population Growth for U.S. Security and Overseas Interests.* It was elaborated in 1974 at the request of Henry Kissinger, then Secretary of State, and was made public 15 years later. We have drawn attention to this report in DTL 85. This same report provided the occasion of an excellent dossier on demography that appeared in *Le Temps de l'Eglise* no. 8, (April 1993) 28-43.

[13] We will content ourselves with mentioning a few documents more recent than the *Kissinger Report*: Gerald O. Barney (ed.), *Global 2000. The Report to the President*, with a Foreword by Jimmy Carter (Arlington: Seven Locks Press, 1991 [1st ed. in 1980]); Shanti Conly, J. Joseph Speidel, Sharon L. Camp, *U.S. Population Assistance: Issues for the 1990s* (Washington: Population Crisis Committee [today; Population Action International], 1991); Office of Population, Bureau for Research and Development, *User's Guide to the Office of Population*, January 1993 (Washington: Agency for International Development, 1993). See also the statement presented by Timothy Wirth on May 11, 1993, to the second committee preparing for the International Conference in Cairo (Sept. 5-13, 1994) on population and development. This text was distributed as a press release by the US Mission to the United Nations Organization and bears the no. 63-93). Betsy Hartmann devoted a remarkably documented article on these questions: "Population Control as Foreign Policy," *Covert Action*, no. 39 (Winter 1991-1992) 26-30.

[14] On this synthetic index see the exemplary work of Gerard-François Dumont, *Démographie. Analyse des populations et démographie économique* (Paaris: Ed. Dunod, 1992) 129 f.

[15] See especially Gerard-François Dumont, *La population de la France en 1992* (Paris: Assoc. pour la Recherche et l'Information Démographiques, March 1993 (cf. question 2).

[16] See *Eurostat. Statistiques démographiques* (Luxembourg-Brussels: l'Office statistique des Communautés européennes, 1993) doc. 3A; cf. p. XLII.

[17] Guy Herzlich, "Quand l'Est se 'depeuple'," *Le Monde*, Nov. 9, 1993.

[18] See *World Population Data Sheet of the Population Reference Bureau* (Washington, 1993)

[19] René *Dumont, L'Utopie ou la mort* (Paris: Seuil, 1973) 49 f., emphasis in the text.

[20] See *World Population. Fundamentals of Growth* (Washington: Population Reference Bureau, 1990).

[21] This concern, "Prevent the Re-emergence of a New Rival," appears in a memorandum of 46 pages prepared by the office of the Secretary of Defense. It was published by the *New York Times* (March 8, 1992) and reported by Barton

Gellman in the *Washington Post* (March 11, 1992) under the title "Keeping the U.S. First. Pentagon would Preclude a Rival Superpower.".

[22] In its issue of March 1993 the *Revue des Deux Mondes* published a dossier on *La Retraite et les retraites*. One should note especially the article of G-F. Dumont on "Le vieillissement, un phénomène social majeur," 104-124.See Alfred Sauvy, "Demographie et refus de voir," in *L'Enjeu démographique*, cited in question 2.

[23] See Alfred Sauvy, "Démographie et refus de voir," in *L'Enjeu démographique*, cited in question 2.

[24] Cf. *Europe Today* (Brussels), no. 111 March 23, 1993, p.8.

[25] According to the *World Population Data Sheet* (Washington: Population Reference Bureau, 1993). On the fertility index see question 85.

[26] On this subject see Bichara Khader, *Le grand Maghreb et l'Europe. Enjeux et perspectives* (Paris: Publishud, 1992).

[27] See for example Pierre Chaunu, *Trois millions d'années* (Paris: Robert Laffont, 1990). This point was also emphasized by Hannah Arendt in *Condition de l'homme moderne* (Paris: Calmann-Levy, 1958, reprinted in 1988) 43.

[28] Cf. DTL 20, 32.

[29] Cf. DTL 51. In *Les spectres de Malthus,* the work cited in question 80, there are studied cases of different countries of the Third World where the demographic situations have been regularly blown out of proportion. Among them figure Togo, New Guinea, Gabon, Ecuador, Ivory Coast, Zaire, Mozambique, Guatemala, Vietnam, Indonesia, Nigeria, Ghana. The case of Bangladesh, often presented as especially "dramatic," is analyzed by B. K. Jahangir and B. Hours (273-278). From this study we see that the numerous poor people of Bangladesh could not be considered as the scapegoats of the misfortunes that have hit this country. They are by and large the victims of corruption, incompetence and the lack of concern for the common good among the leaders.

XII

INTERNATIONAL ORGANIZATIONS

Mention is often made of a campaign of the rich and powerful who   **93.**
devote themselves to limiting the world population of the poor
in order to avoid the obligation of sharing their wealth. Isn't that
a rather gloomy outlook for society and the future of the world?

It is sufficient to read specialized publications, accessible to the public at large, in order to realize the enormous means employed by rich countries to "contain," that is to say curb, the poor population.[1] Some of these same publications also expose, with a pitiless clarity, the scandalous concentration of wealth. Yet, some insist that the South will pose a threat to the North (cf. 82 s., 96).

Without denying the complexity of the problems, we can say that aid to the South is often conditional on acceptance of culturally and morally shocking birth control campaigns.[2] Some even propose that the Third World accept control of its population in exchange for a renegotiation of its debt! The rich decidedly fight with greater ardor against the poor than against poverty (cf. 99)!

Why is it that such publications are so poorly known?   **94.**

What is really dismaying is that people — including politicians — are often so casual when it comes to informing themselves and assessing the information. But that doesn't keep them from speaking out and deciding matters which they make little effort to study.

Can facts be cited to support the contention that this campaign exists? **95.**

We are provided with the first fact by the population fund of the United Nations in its report of 1991.[3] This report recommends widespread distribution of contraceptive methods, whether chemical, mechanical or surgical. The RU 486 is barely mentioned explicitly, but allusion to it is made when it speaks of "new approaches to post-coital contraception" (cf. 96). It is specified that juridical obstacles to its distribution of these methods must be removed.

The second fact comes from the World Health Organization.[4] In a report of 1992, this specialized agency of the United Nations explains why and how it sponsors research on human reproduction.[5] It comes out clearly from this report that the World Health Organization covers with its authority and lends its resources to the effort to distribute widely drugs destined for the control of the population in poor countries. Among these drugs figure preparations that have the effect of provoking early abortions (cf. 96).

No matter how these institutions defend themselves, they really promote the practice of abortion and do it as a method of restricting births (cf. 39).

96. *Is it in this context that the abortive pill RU 486 appears?*
Dr. Baulieu, to whom is attributed the preparation of RU 486, himself admitted that this abortive pill was perfected with the support of the World Health Organization.[6] Moreover, the latter refers to this kind of preparation when it speaks of "post-coital contraception" (cf. 95).

What's more, Dr. Baulieu himself explained that one of the "justifications" for the program of research resulting in RU 486, was the "containing," that is, the restriction of the poor population of the Third World (cf. 76).

97. *Would this mean that the specialized agencies of the United Nations and the United Nations itself are implicated in the anti-birth campaigns in the poor countries?*
The great concern that actually makes its appearance in these international institutions is the creation of a world market (cf. 137).[7] In the planetary market of which some dream, man is no longer simply producer and consumer. He is a product as any other. Man is produced according to the criteria of usefulness, interest, pleasure and solvency (cf. 99).

In some recent publications of these specialized institutions, the United Nations — together with the World Bank[8] -- directed greater and greater attention to the development of this planetary market.[9]

The preferences of this market will determine whether or not a man is admitted to existence or permitted to transmit life.

Man is truly nothing but a solvent individual, capable of consuming and producing.

It is almost unthinkable that an institution of such prestige as the United Nations would offer support to the policies of demographic "containment" involving the practice of abortion. **98.**

According to the Charter agreed upon at San Francisco, we know that the United Nations is an international organization composed of sovereign states. But in this demographic and medical matter, the specialized agencies of the United Nations act more and more as if the UN was a *supranational* organization, that is , one having authority over the sovereign states which are its members.[10]

While carefully avoiding constructing any theory, the UN is in the process of putting into practice a new version of the doctrine of "limited sovereignty." It is little by little abandoning its role as an organ of dialogue and concerted action to transform itself into a directive organ which tends to limit the sovereignty of its members.

Here we have a characteristic *abuse of power*. By way of demographic policies which they discuss, suggest and put into effect, the specialized agencies of the UN induce a change in the very nature of this organization[11]. They tend to make of the UN a supranational authority in the service of the great world market, of a "new world order."[12]

Converging and disquieting indications lead one to believe that the UN, with its specialized agencies, is in the process of becoming an immense machine that manipulates the wealthiest nations of the world, first of all the United States, to put into effect a *world government* for its profit.[13]

Who will profit by this change? **99.**

First of all this change will profit all the wealthy of the entire world: the rich of the developed countries and in the Third World. "Billionaires of the world, unite!"

The wealthy of the entire world have special interests in virtue of which tensions could exist among them. But above all they have *common interests* to defend, and that is why they organize in a sort of new *nomenklatura* to present a common front before the "danger" (in their eyes) presented by the poor everywhere (cf. 70).

Hence, as a conclusion to a tragic confusion, instead of attacking poverty — something that would require sacrifice on their part — they take it out on the poor (cf. 83, 93, 103).

100. *Is this change profitable to certain particular nations?*

The report of the National Security Council prepared in 1970 under the direction of Henry Kissinger, offers some disturbing insights on this point (cf. 84). Kept secret until 1989, this report estimates that it is indispensable to the security of the United States to establish a policy of demographic control in the countries of the Third World (cf. 137). Alongside the pill and sterilization, mention is also made of abortion (cf. 101).

Moreover the report subtly remarks:

And the US can help to minimize charges of an imperialist motivation behind its support of population activities by repeatedly asserting that such support derives from a concern with

a) the right of the individual couple to determine freely and responsibly their number and spacing of children and to have information, education, and *means* to do so; and

b) the fundamental social and economic development of poor countries in which rapid population growth is both a contributing cause and a consequence of widespread poverty.[14]

101. *Does the Kissinger Report speak of abortion?*

a) We read clearly in this Report:[15]

While the agencies participating in this study have no specific recommendations to propose on abortion, the following issues are believed important and should be considered in the context of a global population strategy.

ABORTION

1. Worldwide Abortion Practices

Certain facts about abortion need to be appreciated:

—No country has reduced its population growth without resorting to abortion.

—Thirty million pregnancies are estimated to be terminated annually by abortion throughout the world. . . .

[There follows a brief report on various laws about this]

—The abortion statutes of many countries are not strictly enforced. . . . Lack of medical personnel and facilities or conservative attitudes among physicians and hospital administrators may effectively curtail access to abortion, especially for economically or socially deprived women. . . .

2. U.S. legislation and its policies relative to abortion *A.I.D. Program* [North American Agency for International Development]

The predominant part of A.I.D.'s population assistance program has concentrated on contraception or foresight methods. A.I.D. recognized, however, that under developing country conditions foresight methods not only are frequently unavailable but often fail due to ignorance, lack of preparation, misuse and non-use. Because of these latter conditions, increasing numbers of women in the developing world have been resorting to abortion, usually under unsafe and often lethal conditions. Indeed, abortion, legal and illegal, now has become the most widespread fertility control method in use in the world today. Since, in the developing world, the increasingly widespread practice of abortion is conducted often under unsafe conditions, A.I.D. sought through research to reduce health risks and other complications which arise from the illegal and unsafe forms of abortion. One result has been the development of the Menstrual Regulation Kit, a simple, inexpensive, safe and effective means of fertility control; which is easy to use under LDC conditions.

[There follow considerations regarding the restrictions imposed by the American administration of the time on the use of AID funds for abortion. These considerations end as follows:]

A.I.D. funds may continue to be used for research relative to abortion since the Congress specifically chose not to include research among prohibited activities.

One major effect of the amendment and policy determination is that A.I.D. will not be involved in further development or promotion of the Menstrual Regulation Kit. However, other donors or organizations may become interested in promoting with their own funds dissemination of this promising fertility control method[16] . . .

b) This decision of the United States was confirmed in 1993 and expressed with greater clarity by Timothy E. Wirth, the U.S. representative, in the text cited above (cf.84):

President Clinton is deeply committed to placing population among the top international priorities of America. . . . The government of the USA believes that the Cairo Conference [Sept. 5-13, 1994] will be remiss in its duty if it does not develop recommendations and guidelines regarding abortion. Our position consists in supporting reproductive choice, including access to successful abortion.

Would there be a relationship between the demographic policies of **102.** *the US and the change observed in the nature of the UN?*

One should note first of all that most of the recommendations found in the 1991 Report of the United Nations Fund for Population appear already in the document composed in 1974 under the direction of Henry Kissinger (cf. 84, 100). We learn also that A.I.D. has helped private and public organizations to realize effectively family planning programs.

For the US government to go from there to using these diverse organisms to put into practice its program of demographic containment is but a step that some have already taken.[17] Others have gone even further: why, they wonder, should not the US also use toward this end other organisms — such as the World Bank, the United Nation Fund for population, the World Health Organization, and the UN itself — to implement its policies in this domain?

103. *How can it be explained that the Western democracies join forces with the United States to curb the demographic growth of the Third World?*

As is disclosed in the statistics published by the specialized agencies of the UN, the Western democracies have by and large made common cause with the US in effecting a world program for curbing births in the Third World. By doing that those democracies make themselves objective allies of an imperial project the ultimate control of which the US reserves to itself. (cf. 88).[18]

Without doubt, this alliance is explained, in part, by the fact that many of the leaders of the European democracies are unaware, if not of the existence, at least of the significance and breadth of the campaigns.

But this alliance is also explained by the fact that the wealthy of the entire world — including the bourgeoisie of the Third World — believe it to be in their interest to join a common front to curb the "threat" that, in their eyes, the poor pose to their security.[19]

And so, the wealthy believe that their security is the basis of their right, and they retreat from no means at all to protect the citadel of egoism in which they have shut themselves up (cf. 137).

104. *Is the attitude of these rich people shared by all the citizens of the US and the Western democracies?*

In the United States much more than in Europe, the movements for respecting human life are more and more active and organized better and better (cf. 87). Thanks to them there is developing an awareness analogous to what was observed in the nineteenth century regarding the social question. At that time a minority of citizens became sensitive to the undeserved misery of the working class. And in our day an ever greater number of citizens, and consequently politicians, are becoming sensitive to the undeserved contempt of which human life is the victim all over the world.

Both on the national and world level, these groups which have had their consciousness raised organize and make their actions speak loudly. Their effectiveness is heightened remarkably on different levels. On the economic level, these groups have taught the big pharmaceutical firms producing abortive and/or sterilizing drugs that the arm of the boycott was to be taken very seriously. On the political level, these same groups have led the last presidents of the US to cut their governmental subsidies for financing campaigns of abortion in the Third World as well as to appoint to the Supreme Court some judges known for their determination to place law at the service of innocent life. Even President Clinton, who has broken with his predecessors, will have to take these groups more and more into account.

Isn't it inconsistent for Western nations to export abortifacient **105.**
products while continuing to pose as champions of democracy and development?
Western nations, so prompt to pose as "models" to the entire world, must explain once and for all how they can reconcile the double mission they've arrogated to themselves: on the one hand, their posing as champions of aid for development[20] as well as heralds of human rights everywhere and for all in the world, and yet, on the other hand, for the profit of the *establishment,* their medicalizing[21] political, economic and social problems by offering to this same *establishment* an absolute weapon against "undesirables."

In the eyes of the world, this ambiguity mortgages the credibility of the nations concerned. By what right, for example, can a nation which pays for the production of an abortifacient pill always boast about being the paragon of democracy, even the light of the Third World? How can a state that pays for the distribution of this product (or similar ones) still be taken seriously when it claims to "repent" at the memory of its past errors?

In the final analysis, who are really responsible for and are the real **106.**
restorers of contemporary totalitarianism?
This crucial question must finally be raised. For example, we may frankly question the good faith of certain Western gov-

ernments that place at the disposition of Chinese leaders the anti-life weapons of which, all the world knows full well by reason of the political regime in place, Beijing will make wide and coercive use.[22] How can it be doubted that these governments are steeped in totalitarianism and that their leaders' hands are sullied with blood?

Moreover, how can it be doubted that these same governments are further capable of controlling international organizations and using them to impose their peculiar conception of the "new world economic order"[23] (cf. 98)?

107. *When all is said and done, if no action on behalf of human life is undertaken on a worldwide basis, isn't what is emerging a new war?*
For decades the world has been divided into two blocs: we have seen East and West confront each other. This division is not dead, but today it is relegated to second place and supplanted by the North-South confrontation, a war of rich against the poor. In this war actually in progress new weapons are being put to use, in the first place figure biomedical weapons, and their being put to work was "justified" by a biased reading of demographic data. These new weapons must bring about the final solution of the threat of the poor, if not the existence of poverty. That is why wherever contraception does not yield the expected result, people prefer sterilization and abortion.

It is the same in this case as with partners in search of pleasure: the means for impeding procreation must have an effectiveness without fail (cf. 70, 123). That is why abortion and sterilization are inevitably written into the logic of this new and silent war.

108. *Isn't it excessive to speak of war in respect to abortion?*
Traditional wars kill men in view of conquering their territory, to acquire various advantages, to protect interests, to insure free movement, to gain access to resources, etc.

With the liberalization of abortion, to suppress an unborn infant is presented as the condition for other men to live and be happy. They kill, and they make the law say that it is just to kill, because in this way they enable their rights to prevail. Here man is perceived as the obstacle par excellence to the happiness of man. That is why this war is more pitiless than all others — and therefore more murderous. It is the greatest war of history and the most unjust (cf. 122 f., 139). How is it possible for society to escape unscathed from this carnage?[24]

[1] See for example *Inventory of Population Projects in Developing Countries Around the World, 1991-1992* (new York: United Nations Population Fund, 1993).

[2] See for example *Population and the World Bank. Implication from Eight Case Studies* (Washington, D.C.: World Bank, 1992). Regarding Senegal, for example, we read on p. 58 of this publication: The "recommendation [inviting the World Bank to concentrate its aid to supporting the (Senegalese) government in developing a total demographic policy] was accepted and finally executed, making such a policy statement a condition for the release of the second tranche of the third structural adjustment loan." Another consequence of the acceptance of this policy and the role of the World Bank has been "the development of a Human Resources Project for Senegal, approved by the Administrative Council in April 1992. A condition of the negotiation was the lifting of restrictions on the allocation of services for family planning. . . . A condition for approval was the official adoption of the National Program for Family Planning." See also the study of the same World Bank, *Sub-Saharan Africa: From Crisis to Sustainable Growth* (Washington, D.C.: The World Bank, 1989) 6.

[3] Cf. DTL 67.

[4] Cf. DTL 74.

[5] See *Reproductive Health: A Key to a Brighter Future. Biennial Report 1990-1991. Special Anniversary Issue* (Geneva: World Health Organization, 1992).

[6] See Etienne-Emile Baulieu, *Génération Pilule* (Paris: Jacob, 1990). On RU 486 see Janice G. Raymond, Renate Klein, Lynette J. Dumble, *RU 486. Misconceptions, Myths and Morals* (Cambridge, Ma.: Institute on Women and Technology, IWT, 1991).

[7] Cf. DTL 60.

[8] Cf. DTL 58.

[9] Cf. DTL 60; 133.

[10] Cf. DTL 82.

[11] Cf. DTL 79.

[12] Cf. DTL 79.

[13] See for example William F. Jasper, *Global Tyranny—Step by Step. The United Nations and the Emerging New World Order* (Appleton, WI: Western Island Publishers, 1992). Cf. also James Perloff, *The Shadows of Power. The Council on Foreign Relations and the American Decline* (same publisher, 1990).

[14] This quotation comes from p. 115 of the *Report*. See also pp. 22, 101, 117, etc., of the same *Report*. Cf. DTL 85.

[15] On this point see Stephen D. Mumford and Elton Kessel, "Role of Abortion in Control of Global Population Growth," *Clinics in Obstetrics and Gynecology*, 13 (March 1986) 19-31.

[16] These quotations are taken from pp. 182-184 of the *Report* cited in question 84.

[17] For example, see pp. 113 f. 121 f., 150, 159, 164-166. DTL studies in detail the question which we touch on here. This can be completed by reference to William F. Jasper, *Global Tyranny*, cited in note 13.

[18] See James Kurth, "*Hacia el Mundo Posmoderno.*" *Facetas* (February 1993) 8-13; the original English published by National Affairs, Inc., appeared in *The National Interest*, Summer 1992.

[19] See Exodus 1:8-21.

[20] See the incredible book by Graham Hancock, *Lords of Poverty. The Power, Prestige and Corruption of the International Aid Business* (Boston: Atlantic Monthly Press, 1989).

[21] Cf. DTL 157-172.

[22] Cf. the work of J. S. Aird cited at question 125.

[23] Cf. DTL 85 f.; 121-131; 207.

[24] On these questions see Tony Aantrella, *Non à la société dépressive* (Parish: Flammarion, 1993).

PREVENTION—REPRESSION— ADOPTION

Isn't there at least one point on which proponents and adversaries **109.**
  of abortion are in accord?

All are in accord in saying that abortions is always a defeat, somewhat like suicide. Two attitudes are manifest before an act which we know in advance will be a defeat. On the one hand, one can be resigned to the defeat by accepting it or even regulating it. On the other hand, one can arouse common action among men of good will to prevent the defeat (cf. 15). This defeat is in no way fated; it is avoidable.

Instead of repressing abortion, wouldn't it be better to prevent it? **110.**

Certainly it is clear that we must create conditions that will permit all mothers to carry the child they're expecting in the best possible climate. Some legislators have been trying to do this for years by demanding health care, prenatal examinations, lodging, appropriate education, family allotments, etc.

Nevertheless, even the laws which some call repressive because they punish abortion have in the end the same objective: to *prevent* abortions by extending legal protection to the unborn infant (cf. 17).

A comparison with traffic safety is illuminating: public authorities have good reason to organize campaigns to prevent accidents, and these campaigns happily bear fruit. Yet these preventive measures do not dispense them from pursuing reckless drivers, since they place other people in danger.

Don't legislators who liberalize abortion have a preventive role? **111.**

How can anyone deny that it is indispensable to create conditions that dissuade mothers from having recourse to abortion? Nonetheless, legislation that liberalizes abortion is, by its very nature, an incitement (cf. 41). Previous legislation had mostly a preventive function: the threat of a penal sanction had a dissuasive effect (cf. 49). It is reassuring to state that today certain positive measures are contributing toward preventing abortion, especially when they are accompanied by a warm welcome, adoption, appropriate financial help.

Nevertheless, we must say that the laws liberalizing abortion barely preserve the preventive role except as a preliminary, purely formal, if nonexistent interview. We know what goes on: a rendezvous is arranged for doing the abortion (cf. 110).

112. *Is it necessary, then, to maintain a repression of abortion?*

The unborn child needs an effective juridical protection, and it is toward such protection that notable men and women politicians[1] and lawyers[2] are working. It is necessary that the right of every human being to life be guaranteed by law and that violating this right be punished (cf. 110). We must let live and deal harshly with those who prevent others from living.

Nevertheless, if dissuasion is necessary and indispensable, it is also insufficient. Over and above that, we must assist women in distress and even create such conditions so that awaiting a baby will cause the least possible confusion.

We must not confuse the objectives: dissuade and help. Someone once reproached Mother Teresa of Calcutta for not giving enough schooling to the children she took in. "I feed them," she replied; "it's up to you to do the rest." To provide food, to allow them to live: that is our basic task, which, of course, doesn't dispense us from other duties. The problem, then, is not simply to help some infants escape abortion, but to create a society in which all children can be accommodated. We must punish the reckless drivers, but we must also prevent road accidents.

113. *Does adoption offer an "alternative" to abortion?*

a) If a mother doesn't feel she has the power of loving and making her child happy, there are so many couples and women who long to adopt a baby, love it and make it happy. . .

b) Many couples are sad that they cannot have children and desire to adopt them. Besides, many women would resist abortion if they were better informed of the possibilities of leaving their child, from birth on, in the hands of a family that would acknowledge and love it as its own. To make life easier the formalities of adopting and giving up for adoption would contribute then toward preventing abortion, as would the creation of a welcoming mentality for all abandoned children, regardless of their origin.

[1] One should take note of the courageous action of Christine Boutin, a deputy from Yveslines, who illustrates well he work, *Pour la défense de la vie* (Tequi, 1993).
[2] Cf. EPA 27; 51.

THE CHURCH AND CHILDBEARING

What does the Church say about abortion?   **114.**

 Christians should first remember the "golden rule," attested to by all the great moral traditions of humanity[1] and accepted by many of the greatest philosophers.[2] This "golden rule" is reaffirmed and brought to its perfection in the Gospel: "Do not do to others what you would not have them do to you" (cf. 143).[3]

 Christians must also recall that, according to Scripture, murderers will not enter the Kingdom of God.[4]

 Finally, we must realize that abortion is not just one sin among others concerning the respect due human life, but by reason of the extreme weakness of the victim, it is an "abominable crime."[5]

Regarding respect for human life and in particular respect for the   **115.**
life of the unborn, isn't it a fact that many Christians are in
open opposition to the Church?

 Respect for human life is basic to the definition of Christian identity.[6] To recognize the infinite value of every human individual is essential to all Christian morality, whatever its formulation. Recognizing this value is the very *condition for participating in* Christian morality. It's not a question of a choice left to each one's discretion within the Christian ethic. This truth, objectively established, is so to speak the gate to the whole of Christian morality.

Do not some Christians run the risk of being reproached today   **116.**
with the same lack of courage as lamentable as that of some
Christians of former times?

 A day will come — and is not far off — when one will reproach the blindness and silence of some Christians who have become objective allies, or even active accomplices, of those who have declared war on the most feeble (cf. 89). For them, the judgment of history will be more severe than for those condemned at Nuremburg or for the Christians whom the acrid smoke of Dachau did not choke — precisely because nobody, henceforth, can claim ignorance of Nuremburg or Dachau.[7]

117. *The Catholic Church should take into account the evolution of morals and adapt her conception of sin to them.*

Even though the Church pardons sins, she still does not for all that authorize them. Christ Himself gave her the power of pardoning repentant sinners but not to deny the existence of sin. Thank God some sinners acknowledge their sin; there have always been some and they fill the history of the Church.

The new element which the debate on abortion reveals is that at present people deny sin. One denies transgressions of the natural law first (cf. 43) then of the divine law: in declaring good what is evil, man usurps the place of God and substitutes himself for Him (cf. 18, 51).[8] Not only does man fail to see and acknowledge the evil he does, but this evil he declares good for him. God's forgiveness offered to man, then, loses its object. Thus by blinding himself to his fault, man closes himself to the salvation God offers him. Is that not perhaps sinning against the Holy Spirit?

118. *Why does the Church reject contraception?*

It is always of interest carefully to distinguish the problems. The purpose of contraception is to prevent pregnancy effectively; abortion's purpose is to destroy an infant already conceived (cf. 122).

The Church insists that couples must not radically separate sex and procreation because she maintains that conjugal relations are human acts not reducible to mere instinctive conduct. More precisely, the Church does not approve the methods of contraception because these, in a general way, remove from sexuality one of its essential ends. However, at the same time the Church encourages Christians, with the help of grace, to grow in the practice of freedom and responsibility. Sexuality, freedom, responsibility are, then, included in an integral vision of man. Let us acknowledge it: the requirements of the Church are demanding, like the rest of the Gospel.

119. *Must we not carefully distinguish sterilization from contraception through use of hormones?*

a) First of all, we must not lose sight of the fact that many contraceptive products act equally against nidation, that is to say, they are abortifacient (cf. 122). This said, we must admit that most classic contraceptive methods have, in principle, a *temporary effect*, while sterilization is *definitive*, techniques for reversing it being, as we know, very uncertain.[9]

b) But it is precisely the temporary and provisional character of contraception that makes for a special problem. The psychological mechanism that intervenes here is well known to those who are attentive to human behavior. Contraception separates procreation from pleasure, but not, they say, to reject transmission of life definitively, but to delay it. The pleasure is there, with its reproductive potential, but this potential is suspended, and psychologically speaking procreation is *deferred* or *adjourned*.

c) It is one thing for spouses to have recourse to decent means for postponing conception when special circumstances justify this decision; should the occasion arise, it is even a way for them to exercise responsible parenthood. Quite another thing, however, is to maintain a habitual attitude of *deferring* procreation. Such an attitude is not, in effect, without risk, for in practice everyone knows from experience that delaying an action until later can sometimes mean not acting at all. We know, for example, what goes on among university students: some delay for a time their decision to get to work studying for their exams, and they wind up doing so too late.

d) In the matter of contraception, analogous psychological mechanisms intervene. Some young couples separate pleasure and procreation, all the while asserting that they are only deferring the latter. Now as time passes, these couples see developing in themselves a growing perplexity: "Aren't we getting too old to have children?" And as the woman approaches 35, another consideration confirms her doubt: it is explained to her that at her age she runs the risk of producing an abnormal child.

Thus is reduced the period of effective fertility for couples practicing contraception. While a woman's fertility naturally extends from around 15 to 49, the fertile period for couples having recourse to contraception shrinks to a few years and sometimes disappears totally.

Hence, it is evident that making contraception so commonplace is one of the major causes of the demographic collapse of the so-called developed countries.

When you say responsible parenthood you say contraception. But the Church is opposed to contraception. **120.**

The transmission of life associates man and woman with the creative action of God. It is an act of love because it prolongs the act of love made by God who is all Love and therefore totally free. In the eyes of the Church, human sexuality is less instinctive than hedonist morality wants us to think. It is in the domain of freedom and human responsibility; it cannot be delegated to technicians or abandoned to techniques (cf. 122).

121. *The Church makes it necessary for people to have recourse to abortion because she is opposed to contraception.*

The Neomalthusian current has inculcated public opinion with the idea that *contraception* is the same thing as responsible *procreation* or *birth control*. Such an identification proceeds from a scandalous abuse of language.

a) The Church considers responsible paternity and maternity written in God's design.[10] The Church is favorable toward that and that is why she encourages *natural* methods of birth regulation. But the Church rejects the artificial means called contraception. Why?

First of all because — without envisaging here the demographic consequences (cf. 125 f.) — contraception is always engaged in to the prejudice of one or other spouse: sometimes the men (e.g. vasectomy); more often the women (hormone drugs, the IUD, sterilization).[11] Besides, we are forced to assert that, in this regard, in the European community, cows are better protected than women against hormone drugs.

And so, in consequence, contraception, artificial as it is, drives true freedom from the field of human sexuality. But human sexuality is not purely instinctive; it is responsible and controllable.

b) The spouses' determination to avoid procreation by way of contraception, and for even greater reason by sterilization, rests on an implicit dialogue very easy to reconstitute. It all goes this way, as though the husband says to his wife, always the principal one concerned: "My dear, I love you, but not as you are, that is, fertile. I love you on condition that you be infertile, even sterile. You must model yourself according to my desires so that I can take you when I wish." It is actually against this kind of latent [male] understanding that women are beginning to rise up.[12]

c) More briefly, the Church advises couples that they respect that essential link between sexuality and love. This bond supposes duration, that is, mutual involvement and fidelity (cf.

135). Procreation is inscribed in the framework of this mutual project of conjugal life.

What many have difficulty in understanding is that *the Church wants to save freedom* as a dimension constitutive of human life. This liberty cannot be reduced to the absence of physical or moral restraints; it is not an abandonment to the egotistical impulses of unbridled instinct. Freedom is the ability to consent to values (like good or justice) which reason can discover: it is the capacity to open oneself to another, to love.

The least we can expect of people is to acknowledge that the Church's position is coherent and that it takes seriously man's freedom and responsibility as well as the corporeal dimension of human love.

Isn't effective contraception the best way to avoid abortion? 122.

a) Promoters of abortion have sold public opinion on the idea that prevention of abortion depends on contraception. But the habit of contraception engenders an abortion mentality: if the pill fails, one can easily turn to abortion to repair the "damage."

That fact is both recognized and entirely comprehensible.[13] The contraceptive mentality, in effect, consists of totally separating, in human sexual relations, the *unitive* end, that is, the happiness of the spouses, and the *procreative* end, that is, the transmission of life. It results from the fact that, on the one hand physical union is perceived as a good to be desired and on the other procreation is a risk to be avoided, or an evil to be ruled out (cf. 70, 123).

The total separation of sexual union and fertility, namely contraception, is presented as the greatest victory of woman in search of liberation (cf. 19). Now we must take into account that contraception is of no interest unless it is totally certain. In the contraceptive mentality, this separation has to be as effective and certain as possible. Whence derive two consequences: first of all, the responsibility of sexual conduct and of its consequences — the transmission of life — is left to a technique (cf. 120); and secondly, in case of contraceptive failure, one turns to abortion to save the day.

b) However, the gravest fact that we must point out now is that contraception is becoming more and more identified with abortion.[14] Actually, many of the present pills have the ability to produce three distinct effects:

—The first is contraceptive: it prevents the fertilization of the ovum.

—The second is the effect of a barrier: by modifying the composition of the cervical mucus, the "contraceptive" substance prevents the spermatozoa from entering into the uterus and from there into the fallopian tube to meet the ovum.

—The third is anti-nesting (or "contragestive"): it induces a premature evacuation of the uterus, abortion.

The first two effects are preventive: they go to work beforehand by preventing contraception. The third is posterior, acting after the fact: it destroys the being conceived. But for evident physiological reasons only one of these effects is produced. Sometimes the pill acts a priori; sometimes it acts a posteriori. Either the conception has not taken place, and so the effect is preventive; or conception has taken place and the effect is antinidatory or "contragestive." In any case, we have no way of knowing exactly what takes place.

What results, from the moral point of view, is that the woman, not ever truly knowing what is going on within her, finds herself totally deprived of all moral responsibility, both as regards the fetus which she might have already conceived and as regards her spouse. Total effectiveness joined to the total ignorance in which she finds herself signals her total alienation: she is the object of a determined, ruthless chemical process.

c) In conclusion, one isn't logical when he asserts that he is for contraception and against abortion, since many of the drugs presented as contraceptive are also, if need be, abortifacient. It follows that, in order to get rid of the scourge of abortion, we must abandon contraception and promote the natural methods that favor responsible parenthood.

123. *What consequences are entailed by the separation of sex from procreation in the conjugal union?*

The radical separation of the two ends of conjugal union entails two consequences. First of all, it imperils the very existence of the family cell, notably in favoring free love before marriage. Then, bit by bit, it leads to a state of mind that rejects life and is even haunted by death (cf. 142 f.). Since procreation is an *evil* to be avoided at any price, inevitably one must put to death the one who becomes an obstacle to the sole *good* spouses seek in the conjugal act: carnal union with the pleasure linked to it (cf. 107, 122).

[1] "What you hold as detestable do not do unto your neighbor" (Judaic tradition); "The summary of duty: do not do unto others what, in your mind, would bring you evil" (Hindu tradition); "Do not wound others in such a way as to wound yourself" (Buddhist tradition); "Do not do unto others what you do not want them to do to you" (Confucian tradition); "None of you is a believer if he does not desire for his brother what he desires for himself" (Islamic tradition), etc. Cf. A. Fossion, *Passion de Dieu, Passion de l'homme* (Brussels: De Boeck, 1985) 22.

[2] In philosophy, the "golden rule" is at the center of Kantian morality (1724-1804): "Act in such a way as to treat humanity, both in your person as in the person of all others, always at the same time, as an end and never simply as a means." And, as in all the great moral traditions of humanity, Kant sets in relief the universal scope of this rule: "Perform no action except according to such a maxim that will also imply its being a universal law, such only, then, that the will may be considered itself as constituting, through its maxim, universal legislation at the same time." Cf. Emmanuel Kant, *Fondement de la métaphysique des moeurs* (Paris: Delagrave, 1959) 150 f. and 159.

[3] See, for example, Mt 5:38 ff; 7:12 ff; 22:34. Lk 6:31; Jn 13:34 f.

[4] Cf. Gn 4:10; Ex 20:13; Dt 5:17; Rm 1:29-32; Jn 8:13:34; 1 Jn 3:12-15; Ap 21:8; 22:15.

[5] Cf. *Gaudium et Spes* 51; Canon 1398. The teaching of the Church on abortion is explained in the *Catechism of the Catholic Church* 2270-2275.

[6] This thesis has been masterfully explained by Jean-Marie Hennaux, *Le droit de l'homme à la vie, de la conception à la naissance* (Brussels, Ed. de l'Institut d'Etudes Théologiques, 1993).

[7] See EPA 72.

[8] Cf. EPA 33; 62; 91.

[9] On the psychological aspects of the problems touched upon in this question, see Marie-Magdalene Chatel, *Malaise dans la procréation* (Paris: Albin Michel, 1993).

[10] See *Gaudium et Spes* no. 50 f; Donum Vitae no. 5.

[11] Cf. DTL 307

[12] Cf. A-M. de Vilaine, L. Gavarini, M. Le Coadic (eds.), *Maternité en mouvement. Les femmes, la reproduction et les hommes de science* (Montreal: Saint-Martin, 1986).

[13] Cf. EPA 81; 166-168.

[14] Cf. DTL 76 f.

XV

THE CHURCH
AND DEMOGRAPHY

In what way does the contraception practiced by some couples have **124.**
a political dimension? Isn't it a purely private affair?

a) What is politically worrisome is that the radical separation of sex from procreation allows for the intervention of a third
party — for example, a doctor, whether ordered to do so or not
— in the most intimate interpersonal relationship. Control over
the sexual conduct of spouses, that is to say fertility, risks being
transferred to a new class of technocrats or to the state. Alas, examples from China and Vietnam are only too well known, but
people neglect to reflect on them, They also neglect to reflect on
other examples just as disturbing like that of Brazil,[1]

b) Also our society is witnessing two new forms of *alienation.*

Many children are without parents as well as parents without children (cf. 22). Infants born outside of wedlock, of the
same mother but of different fathers, are found mainly in many
Latin American countries. Deprived of the affection of a family,
they become delinquents, drug "dealers," criminals and prosti-
tutes. This is the drama of the street urchins. If we but observe
that children born outside of marriage are the expression of a
significant aspect of demographic phenomena in the Third
World, then it becomes all the more urgent for us to work at reaf-
firming the value of the family.

On the other hand, if it is not rare that children are alienated from their parents, it is becoming more and more frequent
that spouses are *deprived* of the natural result of their conduct
which is procreation. We are witnessing the dawn of the very reverse of the situation denounced by Marx. For him, in effect, the
proles, or offspring, is the sole riches of the proletariat of which

they weren't deprived. The proletariat described by Marx was deprived, not of children, but of the product of their labor.[2] Now couples of the twenty-first century run the risk of being alienated from their very offspring (cf. 132).

125. *With her morality, doesn't the Church have a heavy responsibility for the world's demographic growth?*

a) First of all, we must remark that countries like India and China, where the demographic situation is — they say— serious and complex, are not suffocating under the influence of the Church or Christian morality.[3] Indira Gandhi suffered a resounding electoral defeat in 1977 because together with her son Sanjay she wanted to impose anti-life measures on the Indians, notably obligatory sterilization.[4] Indians saw the measures as intolerable because inhuman, and they didn't have need of the Church to make this discovery.

b) Moreover, the Church does not deny in any way the existence of world demographic problems; she herself says that they must be seriously examined (cf. 82, 85, 132). But what the Church affirms, above all, is that the problems occasioned as much by demographic growth as by its implosion are first of all of a moral nature. More precisely, their solution is made difficult by reason of the "structures of sin," which bring about innumerable distortions in the process of development. It is this assertion that bothers people, and they reject it.

For the Church, under-development and poverty have their source in egoism, materialism, injustice, incompetence, laziness, corruption, imbalance in distribution of wealth, bad organization, etc. But the Church adds right away: there are solutions to these problems, and these solutions are called the rights of man, respect, justice, peace, solidarity, love.

126. *Why do so many reject the Church's message about misery in the Third World?*

Faced with the poor, the wealthy have a bad conscience and, according to a classical process, they are in search of a scapegoat to explain all of the dysfunction in present-day society.

They therefore believe the poor are responsible for their poverty (cf. 83). At the same time, the wealthy are closed to any discussion that would lead them to see that one of the major causes of misery is found in the hardness of their heart. And the tragedy is that they refuse to change their way of life.

127. *Doesn't the conjugal morality of the Church favor having children?*

The conjugal morality of the Church is basically open to welcoming life, but that does not mean that she is a dyed-in-the-wool promoter of births at any cost (cf. 121). In her constant teaching, the Church recommends *responsible* parenthood (cf. 130). The Church doesn't ask that Christians have as many children as possible, but she does ask that Christians have as many children as they are reasonably and generously able to welcome and raise in the circumstances in which life has placed them.[5]

128. *According to some specialists, the Church's position in the matter of contraception and demography is going to cause dramatic consequences — notably famine.*

According to the very information given out by the Food and Agriculture Organization and the UN Fund for Population, whose actions to control demography are well known, there is actually enough food to feed the planet (cf. 80, 82, 102). The problem is neither demographic nor agronomic; it is a moral, political and organizational in nature (cf. 92).

That doesn't prevent some alarmist agronomists and demographers from advocating "permits to procreate," as they exist in China. When one remarks that this idea was already proposed by Hitler in Mein Kampf, there are some people who get furious. Yet that is the truth, and it would be better to draw the right conclusions. . .

129. *Why would one institute "permits to procreate" in wealthy countries where the birth rate is suffering such a disquieting decline?*

The answer to this question is given with all clarity by the promoters of demographic planning. What in substance do they say? First of all, abortion should be allowed; even a permit should be required in order to live in wealthy countries (cf. 143). Then, following the example of these countries, one would introduce these practices and make them widespread in the countries of the Third World.[6] Why, in any case, should a country that doesn't hesitate to kill its own children hesitate to kill those of others (cf. 86, 103)?

That in the long run these practices will prove suicidal for the wealthy countries themselves seems hardly to bother them. . . Destined for the Third World, these suicidal campaigns wind up turning against the wealthy countries that began them (cf. 86). This boomerang effect will have repercussions in the Third World itself, where there are better educated minorities (more precious therefore for stimulating development) which have access to the anti-birth armory.

130. *Where do we find the Church's teaching on population? Isn't it contained in her pro-birth conjugal morality?*

What the Church says about the demographic question is found above all in her *social doctrine*, which on this point is particularly illuminated by conjugal morality.[7] For the rest, as we have explained (cf. 23), this conjugal morality is oriented toward responsible parenthood.

Nevertheless, many do not realize that Christian social morality is as demanding as the conjugal morality of the Church.[8] Now, what the Church says in her social doctrine, first of all, is that it is not man who is made for the market, but the market is made for man. Man's life cannot be organized principally or even exclusively in view of the demands of the market as it is understood in liberal ideology.

The Church adds that the problems of development and population result from the general egoism of those who refuse to put their life-style on trial, refuse to convert (cf. 126), and thence are led to call into question the right of the most destitute to live (cf. 137).

131. *Doesn't the Church completely neglect the demographic problems when she proclaims her beautiful principles concerning development?*

The Church says that it is inadmissible, in studying development, to exalt the importance of the demographic factor and to act on it first of all without wishing to change the other factors in depth. It is inadmissible that one is so much less disposed to touch the other parameters. What parameters, for example? The excessive expense for weapons and the plethora of bureaucracies; insufficient funds for territorial management, agriculture, health; pathetic, laughable attempts at education. Other considerations aside, the Gulf War, for example, cost a billion dollars a day.

132. *In this question of demography, aren't Catholic moralists in bad faith? In effect, they say that development entails a drop in the birth rate, but they hide the fact that this decline in the birth rate is obtained, in developed countries, by methods condemned by the Church.*

a) It is true that in part the birth rate is regressing in the wealthy countries due to methods condemned by the Church. The best proof that these techniques are evil and that the Church has the right and duty to condemn them is precisely that the countries in which they are used have fallen below the rate of fertility needed for replacement of their population.[9] In the rich countries this rate is 2.1 children per woman of childbearing age (cf. 85). One can easily see that these methods are bad from the results to which they lead. If they continue to be applied as they have been, the nations which use them on a grand scale will disappear.[10] From 1960 to 1980 the birth rate among women of childbearing age went from 2.57 to 1.60 in Belgium. In France it went from 2.56 to 1.62, despite the significant immigration. In turn, the latter poses different problems.[11] Is it an exaggeration, then, to speak of the suicide of a nation?

Whether one wants to listen to the Church or not when she condemns these methods, the fact remains, and attention better be paid to it, they are ravaging the countries in which they are widely used. They are not good, therefore.

b) On the other hand, it is entirely correct to say that in countries where there is absolutely no effective protection for the poor, aggravated poverty increases in a formidable way the desire to have numerous children, *because that is the sole means of survival*. All who work the earth know that poor people often say: "There will be at least one or other of my children to feed and care for me when I get old."

How can one say the Church is wrong? She says that in societies that do not protect the poor strata of the population, it is poverty itself that drives one to this way of surviving pinned to the affection of a child. The deep and really *unique* reason that inspires this conduct — one which Marx perfectly identified — is that the child is the sole riches of the poor (cf. 124). To have a lot of children is the only recourse the poor have for surviving in the future.

When there is no social security, who will feed the aged if not their children. And since these children are themselves victims of a very elevated mortality rate because they are badly cared for and don't have enough to eat, they have to make quite an effort to survive.

Hence, it is perfectly logical to say that when one fights effectively against poverty, this search for assurance — from offspring — loses its reasonableness. This new situation, then, diminishes the desire and need for numerous descendants.

c) Catholic moralists, then, have no reason to hide behind such a situation. They must, on the contrary, denounce it and contribute towards its remedy. To those who ask approval of their "modern" methods, the Church recommends: *"Take note of where your actions are leading you. You were told that these meth-*

ods were evil; see, nature itself is showing you that you're doing evil to yourselves and to others."

d) However, the Church has never pretended that it is easy to reach a regulation of births, in a given population, by honorable methods (cf. 121). She emphasizes, nevertheless, a regularly hidden fact: namely that once one uses dishonorable and inhuman methods, one is headed for catastrophe. Either it doesn't work, or one kills oneself.

We must end by wondering whether the reproach of hypocrisy shouldn't be sent to another address.

133. *Isn't it dreaming to imagine that natural methods can be widely distributed and used?*

For the Church, instruction in natural methods of birth control must be made part of the basic education to which every man and woman has the right (cf. 100, 110). It is by wide distribution of these methods that we can hope to arrive at a balanced birth rate with respect for the specific character of human sexuality, of persons and of spouses.

The easy means now spread by our consumerist society have the characteristic of unleashing a catastrophic demographic upheaval (cf. 132) and of being an assault against the spouses who use them (cf. 121). Moreover, as actual practice confirms, these easy means expose human reproduction to an imperative of planning that deprives the couple of their responsible liberty.

It is disquieting to see that China, a contrary major example of a developing country and bastion of an out-of-date totalitarianism, is cited with praise by Western contraceptors for the barbarous effectiveness of its anti-life campaigns (cf. 124, 128).

134. *Isn't it out of naïveté, if a provocative spirit, on the part of Christians to advocate recourse to natural methods?*

The world situation, in which violence is at work under different forms,[12] impels Christians to study, to refine and to make better known the natural methods for mastering fertility.[13] These have the immense advantage of being less "aggressive" and less exacting on the woman (cf. 16, 121). Consequently, they respect better the spouses' harmony. Moreover, they predispose couples to exercise their responsible freedom in political and economic society.[14]

These natural methods, too often misunderstood and discredited, have, besides, proven their ability effectively to make population growth bend exactly where the problem arises. Mother Teresa received from Rajiv Gandhi one of the highest distinctions of India because, in Calcutta, she had succeeded where the technicians of "modern contraception" had failed (cf. 125).

Discussions concerning natural methods refer us, then, to an in- **135.**
depth reflection on human development?

If the ideal of human development is conceived like a race for consumerism and ease, the so-called "modern" methods of contraception are certainly going to be understood in this sense (cf. 20).

a) Nevertheless, just as we have already brought out, these methods have had and have as their result a catastrophic fall in the birth rate and an aging of the population (cf. 132). The effects resulting from them are already being felt in developed countries and are beginning to be perceptible in some countries of the Third World. This demographic plunge and the aging of the population will inevitably create grave difficulties for the next generations notably of a social and economic order. They will further aggravate the tensions occasioned by emigration.

b) On the other hand, if the ideal of development is seen rather as the *education of people to responsibility*, fraternity, generosity, then mastery of fertility can very well be achieved without recourse to methods condemned by the Church (cf. 134).

c) Hence, mankind has the choice between responsible means and violent means (cf. 121). The discussion about methods allowed or rejected by the Church leads us, then, to bring up again the problem of the *quality of human development* which leads us once more to the problem of the relationship between the spouses.

What, then, is the heart of the Church's social teaching on **136.**
demography?

All the social teaching of John Paul II is an appeal to the *solidarity* of all men, in space as well as in time. There is enough food (cf. 128), enough resources, enough knowledge, enough know-how to relieve the poor of their misery. But what is needed is the effective will to share and to raise the level of life of the poor in order, consequently, to enable them to alter their fertility.

Furthermore, in the eyes of the Church, the lowering of the birth rate cannot occur except by way of a responsible attitude, and that excludes lies, coercion and violence.[15] For her, the demographic question cannot be resolved except with a respect for the dignity of each human being. Anything resembling a demographic police must be rejected with contempt

137. *Why do the ideologues of demographic security give so much attention to ecological problems?*

In its different formulations, the ideology of demographic security[16] resumes, while modernizing it, the well known doctrine of *living space*. It was in the name of the Aryan race's right (cf. 32) to living space, presumed indispensable, that the Nazi state launched its wars of territorial expansion.

a) There is reason to redouble our guard (cf. 92) when the ideologues of contraception and contragestion accompany their discourses with warnings to people about "the deterioration of the environment" and "the exhaustion of natural resources."[17] Parallel to the discussion on demography, the talk about the ecosystem is regularly called to the rescue of the anti-birth harangues. It risks dissimulating the same motives and being called to "legitimize" the same programs for curbing the poor population.

Just as in the time of Malthus, they tone down the capacity of man to add a "plus"to nature, and they insist that the "human cattle" (cf. 36) be kept within the limits technocrats are employed to define.

b) The powerful people of the entire world put to work here, for their own profit, the doctrine of living space which their precursors invoked in favor of race (cf. 31 f.). However, invoking the right to living space goes further here than at the beginning of the century. In effect, the rich and powerful intend, not only to *preserve* their *present* well-being, but they try to apply in some way to their descendants a preemptive right over natural resources as well as the means to deal with them (cf. 92, 103). Knowing that the poor will not be able to add any value to them, the rich reserve their use in advance. In some way they are purchasing the future.

c) This concept of *living space* allows the US in particular to reinterpret its idea of its frontier.[18] This was understood to mean a constantly moving border reached by explorers. These latter intended to replace the "natives" — sometimes by killing them — in order to enjoy the benefits of the natural resources that, according to them, the "natives were incapable of appropriately exploiting." This *frontier* moved toward the South (where it became the origin of the war of secession) and toward the West; it also moved toward the Southwest by annexing territories belonging to Mexico. But this *frontier* hasn't stopped moving even now, in particular toward the Latin American continent, regarded since Monroe, as the "garden" of the United States. A "garden" whose extension never ends — under reinforced control.

d) The wealthy countries extend their *"preemptive right" to knowledge and know-how* They jealously guard for themselves the important areas. For example, by taking advantage of

GATT, they carefully choose what knowledge they are disposed to share. The US withdrew from UNESCO once it realized that countries of the Third World claimed a "new world order" of information. The US and other wealthy countries know that a large population, *if it is well formed*, is a source of development because it is favorable to exchanges. But how can we forget that all the totalitarian regimes endeavored to impoverish these exchanges, thereby fixing nations in their undeveloped state?

e) Thus we see the close connection that exists between the campaigns to *control human life* and the *conservationist mentality*. The powerful of this world regard their security as the foundation of their rights (cf. 70): not only of their right to control the whole of the world's population, but to control all the resources, including the intellectual resources. Now this obsessive fear about security engenders, in individuals as well as societies, an avarice of a new kind and inhibits creativity. Such avarice consists in invoking the internationalization of human society and the market in order to withdraw from the poor the disposal of their natural resources (cf. 100). The rich and the powerful want to perpetuate the present; they only want foresight in birth control. But it's bad foresight, because by emphasizing that an infant costs, they loose sight of the fact that there will normally come a day when it will bring in money. Like all the avaricious, the rich think of the future as the overcautious consolidation of their present well-being. They refuse to make the least projection, for it would lead them generously to call into question today's practices in the name of a more just world with greater solidarity that we would like to see blossom tomorrow (cf. 136).

[1] Cf. DTL 157. See also Délcio da Fonseca Sobrinho, *Estado e População. Uma história do Planejamento familiar no Brasil*. (Rio de Janerio: Rosa dos Tempos et FNUAP, 1993). On the attitude of the US and of the Brazilian military government, see 91-100. One should finally refer to Carlos Penna Botto, "Explosão demográfica," *Revista maritima brasileira* (Rio de Janeiro) 113 (Jan.-March 1993) 103-113.

[2] Hannah Arendt devoted several remarkable pages to the relationships between work and procreation in the work cited in question 91. See, for example, pp. 133, 152 f.

[3] The case of China has been recently studied by one of the best world specialists in the demography of this country, John S. Aird, *Foreign Assistance to Coercive Family Planning in China. Response to Recent Population Policy in China* [by Terence Hull] (Canberra, 1991).

[4] Cf. the *Britannica Book of the Year, 1978* (Chicago: Encyclopedia Britannica) 434.

[5] Cf. DTL 308.

[6] Cf. DTL 166.

[7] John Paul II's teaching on life given during the first ten years of his pontificate is the object of a collection of over 800 pages! See Giovanni Paolo II, *Dieci anni per la vita*, Giovanni Caprile ed. (Rome: Centro Documentazione e Solidarietà, 1988). See also *Le droit à la vie* (Solesmes 1981) and in the collection "Ce que dit le pape" in Editions du Sarment-Fayard: *De la sexualité à l'amour* (n. 15); *Se préparer au mariage* (n. 7), *L'euthanasie* (n. 11).

[8] This is what John Paul II emphasizes in his encyclical *Veritatis Splendor* 95-101.

[9] Cf. DTL 33 f. See other data at question 85.

[10] On this subject see the forceful Communication à l'Academie des Sciences morales et politiques de Paris presented on Oct. 18, 1993 by Gerard-Francois Dumont under the title *De "l'explosion" à "l'implosion" démographique?*

[11] Cf. *Eurostat* (1993) table E 10, p. 98. According to *Eurostat*'s data, in the report of 1975 nearly seven million less students today attend primary schools in the CE countries." See *Europe Today* n. 111 (March 23, 1992) 1.

[12] Cf. DTL 231-236.

[13] Cf. DTL 170; 306-308. See also Joseph Rötzer, *La régulation naturelle des naissances* (Paris: Mediaspaul, 1987).

[14] Cf. DTL 170-172.

[15] Cf. DTL 308.

[16] Cf. EPA 189-208.

[17] Cf. DTL 57-86.

[18] Cf. Peter Bauer, *The Development Frontier* (Boston: Harvard Press, 1991).

XVI

Resume and Conclusions

Doesn't the decriminalization of abortion and its practical con-   **138.**
sequence, its liberalization, pose serious threats to our society?

The philosopher Simone Weil (1909-1943) wrote to Bernanos: "Once temporal and spiritual authorities have placed a category of human beings beyond those whose life has a price, there is nothing more natural than to kill. When one knows he can kill without risk of punishment or blame, he kills; or at least one surrounds with encouraging smiles those who do kill. If by chance one experiences at first a bit of disgust, he remains silent and soon he smothers it for fear of lacking virility."[1]

Are we not witnessing the execution of a scientific program of social   **139.**
engineering?

The means presently available for destroying human life or for drying up its sources are incomparably more effective than those which the totalitarian fascist, Nazi and communist regimes had at their disposal. The time is rapidly approaching when everyone will be hit, with the lightning of facts, already evident for many, that the great harm now being done by the organizations attacking human life has surpassed by far the deeds of Hitler and Stalin taken together. That's entirely normal, for we are now dealing with genuine *managers* executing a program of *social engineering,* whose object is to program scientifically the destruction of future eventual enemies.

With nearly six billion inhabitants haven't we reached the limits of   **140.**
the earth's capacity?

a) Like "overpopulation," the "sustaining capacity" of the earth is a totally relative notion (cf. 82, 137). The limits of the earth's "sustaining capacity" are strictly *undefinable,* because strictly speaking, they are indefinite: it is impossible to determine them.

Why is it impossible to determine them? Very simply because it is fortunately impossible to assign any limit whatsoever to man's ability to intervene in the world.

Without forcing the paradox, one can say, with the economist Sheldon Richman, in the final analysis there are no natural resources (cf. 92, 137).[2]

b) The Indians in Texas lived for centuries above oil deposits which they didn't know how to exploit. As long as it was simply there, oil was just a thing. It didn't become a natural resource until the moment men took interest in it, and made of it a source of energy and the basis for innumerable chemicals

Titanium, discovered at the end of the eighteenth century, did not become a natural resource until 1947, once its light weight, its hardness and its resistance to corrosion began to be exploited in the aerospace industry and later in surgery. It is one of the most abundant of all the chemicals found in the earth: it is in ninth place. What made it a *natural resource* was the genius of man.

Silicone was discovered at the end of the eighteenth century. After oxygen, it is the most abundant chemical element in the earth, where it is present notably as sand. Traditionally it was used for ceramics, now it is widely employed in metallurgy. However, for decades it has been at the basis of the electronic revolution. More recently still, under the form of fiber optics, it has revolutionized methods of medical diagnosis and telecommunications.

Motor manufacturers are trying to produce airplane motors that consume less gasoline. When they produce a motor that uses 30% less gasoline than even the motor of a preceding generation, they increase the oil reserves all the more.

The wind has been used in Holland for centuries, first of all to dry out the lowlands (the land flooded by the sea) and to grind wheat, then for producing electricity.

Research in agronomy and zootechnics is still progressing (cf. 104, 126). In countries of the Third World, only those holding on to an archaic vision of agriculture and breeding continue to manage the land as though men were cattle (cf. 36) and as though the yield of the soil was condemned to be what it has always been.

C) Japan understood very early on that the primal resource — and as it were the unique resource — of which it could dispose was man. That is why it made — and continues to make — an exemplary effort in education and professional training of its youth.

d) In conclusion, one can say that the principal, even unique resource of man is his intelligence and his free will, by which his resemblance to God is most explicitly manifested. Thanks to these eminent gifts, man has the capacity of constantly ameliorating his relationship to nature, of bringing to its elements additional value, of transforming materials into goods, of better organizing society. It offends his dignity to present man as a consumer predisposed to destroy this surrounding environment, or as a predator programmed to defend his living space.

When all is said and done, must we not stop speaking of overpopulation? **141.**

An American friend of mine with whom I discussed this question arrived at a simple conclusion that merits being shared.[3]

a) What is *overpopulation?* It's the imbalance between the number of men and the volume of goods that are available. What is *poverty?* It is the imbalance between the number of men and the volume of available goods. The words "overpopulation" and poverty" have an identical meaning every time they're used to describe the same social situation. They imply, however, very different judgments. In fact, the world "overpopulation" has become a *pejorative* term to designate "poverty."

b) When one thinks of the situation in "poor countries," he is inclined to help them produce more goods and distribute them better. What is recommended is educational and economic development as well as social justice (cf. 115).

But when one speaks of these same countries in terms of "overpopulation," the solution proposed — and one had the effrontery to call it "aid"! — consists in sterilizing people, making the mother have abortions, because the men and women are regarded as the cause of the social problems they experience (cf. 83). And that dispenses one from questioning their living conditions.

c) When we speak of "poor people," our hearts are moved; we rise up against the situations of injustice of which the poor are victims; we mobilize and want to express our solidarity (cf. 63).

When we speak of "overpopulation," however, the rich feel that their security is threatened (cf. 70, 137). Elementary concern for justice melts like snow before the sun. Instead of wanting to express our solidarity (cf. 10), we persuade ourselves — with a big dose of bad faith — and we persuade the unfortunate people, by trapping them in their inability to judge, that it's "for their welfare and that of human society" that they must accept organized contraception, sterilization en masse and abortion (cf. 69, 80).

Briefly, more concerned for their security than for solidarity, the wealthy invoke "overpopulation" to "justify" the coercion practiced on the poor.

142. *Is the "culture of death" a characteristic of our century?*

a) During the twentieth century ideologies have been spread that see reason incarnate in the State, in the "super-race," in the Party (cf. 67-69). The State, for example, "had reason" to demand total submission of individuals, and it was "reasonable" for the individuals to submit totally to the State which transcended them. Regarding themselves as incarnating reason, the State, the Race or the Party was founded to say who would live or must die: the State, the Race or the Party was master of life and death (cf. 60). The henchmen of the Nazi regime, for example, displayed a death's head on their uniform; it was a summary of their program. The regime, of which they were both the instrument and expression, expected them to disregard their own lives by putting themselves unconditionally at the disposal of the State and scorn the lives of others as well.

The totalitarian ideologies regarding the State, the Race and the Party as sacred presented this common point that they taught individuals to liberate themselves from all material and intellectual attachments, and from all moral reference. They were beyond good and evil (cf. 32, 51), and the service of the State, the Race and the Party required that the individual be disposed to empty himself unto death. To expose my life to death and to inflict death on others was thus the climactic expression of sovereign liberty *at the service of the Cause:* that is the State, the Race or the Party.

Hegel, of whom we are going to speak, was at once the source and interpretative key of these ideologies and of the neo-liberal ideology.[4]

b) In the present paroxysms of expression, the neo-liberal current cannot be understood unless it is situated in the funeral cortege of totalitarian ideologies that the twentieth century wanted to deify. For this new ideological current, in effect, the affirmation par excellence of the sovereign liberty of the individual is found in unrestrained consumerism, that is, in the possibility of wasting, which means to destroy without having to render an account to anybody. To consume, to waste is also a way of freeing oneself from all material attachment, from all moral or juridical reference. It is a way of affirming the sovereignty of the Ego.

Now, as we have seen this affirmation of the sovereignty of the Ego leads the individual to want to dispose of the life of others (cf. 8 f., 70). I dispose of the life of the infant or of the handicapped, or of the bedridden old person, or of the poor, if they are of no use to me. On the other hand, I will produce a child if the social security reserves are gone when I come to the age of retiring (cf. 30). I will admit the poor to existence, if by means of their low salaries they permit me to consume and waste, that is, to affirm me as master (cf. 97).

c) We are approaching bit by bit the possible limit of this evolution. It is attested to by the slide of the aggressive trend, described above, to the suicidal drift observed in wealthy Western society (cf. 129). The latter wished to affirm its sovereign liberty in two complementary fashions. It burns its past by making it impossible for lack of men to inherit it and thus ends the transmission of its handed on patrimony (cf. 77, 91). It burns its future by refusing to people it and by sacrificing it totally to the present (cf. 137).

The individuals characteristic of this society break the natural solidarity (cf. 63), synchronic (between individuals and contemporary societies) and diachronic (between individuals or societies linked by generations), by reason of the fact that they don't have to answer to anyone but themselves for their own life and death. They, therefore, provide themselves with institutions and "rights" in accord with the affirmation of what they regard as the sovereign expression of their liberty: to give death and even to give themselves to death.

Georges Bataille, who surpasses Sade on this point, perfectly sums up this *nihilism:* "Life was the search for pleasure, and pleasure was proportional to the destruction of life. Said in another way, life attained its highest degree of intensity in a negation of its principle."[5]

d) It is, then, by the same "culture of death" that we explain, not only the dismal regimes our century has known, but also the obstinate insistence on legalizing abortion and euthanasia as well as making mass sterilization commonplace. The spread of AIDs finds therein one of its most evident explanations. The common root of all these manifestations of the "culture of death" is nihilism (cf. 32), itself based on the revolt against finitude.[6] Men cause death and give themselves over to death because they believe it impossible for the desire for the beyond to be fulfilled, a desire nonetheless finely engraven on their souls. And so they believe themselves freed from this desire by the sovereign enjoyment they seek in death. Now, death thus conceived is in reality the supreme expression of despair. According to the new liberal ideology, it is, in the final analysis, this despair that must be shared by the poor if they are to be subdued.

Is there a task more exalting and joyous, especially for Christians, than to show why we must prefer *the choice of life?*[7]

143. *Instead of being part of the "culture of death," isn't genetic manipulation oriented to the service of life?*

a) Different projects or proposals of law concerning genetic manipulation are now being discussed. One thing in these discussions is immediately striking: appeal is made once again to the tactic of *dispensation* (cf. 3): they quibble in order to define the condition under which they can evade the law which pretends to assure protection to the embryo.

On the level of principles, these discussions do not differ fundamentally from those that preceded the legalization of abortion. In any case, they attest, more clearly than ever, the fascination that the culture of death exercises. The right of a human being to life, from its most secret beginnings, is more and more dependent on a *procedural* decision (cf. 61). This decision is taken by laboratory technicians disposed to regard as moral all possible manipulations.

The fascination with death appears here in all its aspects. From its embryonic stage, the human individual is not considered to have any dignity of himself; he doesn't command respect. This denied acknowledgment operates, first of all, on the practical level then on the theoretical — for the practitioners are anxious to fabricate legitimizing theories. From its most hidden origins, the life of the human being is under a suspended sentence; the embryo is totally disposable (cf. 34-38). As Professor Jerome Lejune remarked, the embryo is treated like a product of the human body; it is placed on the same level as the egg or spermatozoa, though it is already a newly produced human being.

The future of this being is *hypothetical* in the strict sense of the word: the eventual outcome of this future is totally *subordinated to the quality* recognized or not in the embryo or to the usefulness it offers.

b) This double criterion — quality, usefulness — is one of the major expressions of the morality of lord, that is , of a master before his slave (cf. 32, 142). The master believes that, because he is capable of arousing life, he is justified in dealing death. This lordly morality, whose Hegelian source we have noted (cf. 142), considers the supreme expression of the liberty of the finite being who is man to consist in exercising a mastery as total as possible over life and death.

This "lordly mastery" over life is expressed in various ways. First of all it gives rise to a *cellular cannibalism*, a condition preliminary to reconstruction by the manipulator of a being who will be, in rigorous terms, the incarnation of his very own project. Then it gives rise to a *histological cannibalism* which — while awaiting other uses — has recourse to the brain tissue of aborted fetuses, which is grafted, for example, on to patients suffering from Parkinson's disease. It still gives rise to *"academic"* or *"scientific" cannibalism* in this sense that the human being will be manipulated, ground up, immolated on the altar of scientific research — all done under the aegis of academic freedom totally liberated from any moral reference and not having to answer to anybody. Finally, it gives rise to a *technicalized eugenicism,* alongside of which the eugenicism of history was but pathetic mumbling. This eugenicism, with its frightening performance, opens to the practitioners of ultraNaziism (cf. 75) the horizon of a reckless scientific segregation. In effect, the typology of selection and discrimination is totally at the discretion of the manipulators.

Can we foresee the consequences of these manipulations and the **144.** *legislation attempting to legitimize them?*

At least two terrible consequences are the foreseen price of these manipulations and their "justifications." We will indicate the following two.

a) The first is that the medical profession in its entirety is more and more subjected to pressures that will transform doctors insidiously into artisans of death. Works of death: that is already what innumerable gynecologists are producing who practice abortion and participate in campaigns of contraception; that is already what surgeons are producing who perform sterilizations; that is already what internists, anesthetists and cancer specialists are producing when they practice euthanasia. Work of death: the genetic manipulators are already implicated in that more and more. In brief, the culture of death is about to cause an appreciable part of the medical profession to topple over into the camp of the enemies of life (cf. 75). If the medical world — and with it, the infirmaries and all the health workers — does not recover, if it does not withdraw from this bewitching spiral, suspicion will affect the whole medical profession; the most precious capital of the profession —confidence —will be definitively ruined. Deprived of all effective legal protection, the weakest of human beings — all categories confused — will also be deprived of all reliable medical aid.

b) The second consequence is, however, the most dramatic that we can imagine. Because the culture of death underlies them, genetic manipulations and the laws pretending to lend their support result, not only in the destruction of life, but also in the destruction of love and the family, the foyer of both. Here we find renewed an anti-family tradition that goes back all the way to Frederick Engels. The logic of these manipulations is, in effect, very simple, and its "lordly" character is going to appear still again. The deep motivation from which emanates the will to manipulate can be expressed in these terms: "I am strong enough, powerful enough, not to need anyone else to be myself. I don't have, then, any reason to run the risk of discovering that I am poor — either in the eyes of others or my own. Why, then, should I risk the adventure of loving and being loved? All true love that I might show to others or which I might experience from others would be an unbearable mark of weakness and poverty, the supreme sign of my finiteness — exactly what I want to reject and deny. And so, since I have given myself the power, I will dispose of others to my liking or fashion them to my convenience, according to the criteria of quality that is appropriate to me and the usefulness that I define."

Thus we have the spiraling chain with which the culture of death binds human society.

Before such a challenge, the like of which history knows no precedent, there is only one response: welcome joyously the daily experience of our poverty, for it, if accepted, becomes the anchorage for our hope. Paradoxically, it is on this condition that we are able to love and opens ourselves to love, to welcome and be welcomed. This is the price of our being able to rediscover the very thing that seems to create such fear in many of our contemporaries: tenderness.

Briefly, on the whole, rather than the culture of death, why not risk the *culture of life?*

In many of the reasons given, aren't there special reasons that impel 145.
  Christians to promote respect for life?

Christian morality subscribes without reserve to the "golden rule" of all the world: "Do not do unto others what you would not have them do to you" (cf. 59, 114).

Furthermore, the Christian doesn't ask himself who is worthy of being his neighbor; he asks himself instead how can he make another his neighbor (cf. Lk 10: 25-37).

Finally, the Christian believes that the forces of evil are at work in the world, and it was to save all men that Jesus came into the world. By their violence, the campaigns for abortion and euthanasia aim at and reach man, but they also aim at God. Powerless to destroy God, the forces of evil want to destroy man who is the living image of God from the beginning to the end of his life. For the Christian, all men have received existence from the same God and *that is why* they are brothers. Consequently, *every* man must be, not only respected, but loved, because he expresses something of the goodness and beauty of God, and because he is destined to eternal life.

Finally, would human life be a sign of hope for all men? 146.

We will let Hannah Arendt, one of the greatest political philosophers of our time. reply to this last question.[8]

The miracle that saves the world, the domain of human affairs, from normal, "natural" ruin, is finally the fact of birth, in which is rooted ontologically the faculty to act. In other words it's the birth of new men, the fact that they begin anew, the action they are capable of by right of birth. Only the total experience of this capacity can bestow on human affairs faith and hope, these two essential characteristics of existence which Greek antiquity completely misunderstood, setting aside vowed faith in which they saw a very rare and negligible virtue, and ranking hope among the number of pernicious illusions of Pandora's box. It is this hope and faith in the world which have found, without doubt, their most succinct and glorious expression in the little phrase of the Gospel announcing the "good news": "A child is born to us."

---

[1] Cited, along with many other interesting texts, by Jacques Verhagen in the rich collection he organized on *Licéité en droit positif et réferences légales aux valeurs* (Brussels: Bruylant, 1982) 166.

[2] Cf. Sheldon Richman, "Population is no Threat to Progress," *Freedom Daily* (Washington, D.C.) July 1993, 18-23.

3 Cf. Michael Schwartz, "Overpopulation and the War on the Poor," manuscript of talk given at the Third InternationalConference of the Family of the Americas Foundation in Caracas, Venezuela, Oct, 1985.

4 To understand the influence of Hegel on these ideologies, one can consult Alexandre Kojève, *Introduction à la lecture de Hegel* (Paris: Gallimard, 1968), esp. 529-575 devoted to "L'idée de la mort dans la philosophie de Hegel." There we read: "Acceptance of death without reserve, or of human finiteness aware of itself, is the ultimate source of Hegelian thought. . . . According to this thought, it is by voluntarily accepting the danger of death in a fight for prestige that man appears in the natural world for the first time; and it is by resigning himself to death and revealing it in his discourse that man finally arrives at the absolute Savior or Wisdom and thus achieves History. For it is in taking the idea of death as his point of departure that Hegel elaborates his 'absolute' science or philosophy, which is alone capable of taking philosophical account of the fact of existence in the world of a finite being conscious of its finiteness and sometimes disposing of it as he pleases" (cf. p. 540).

5 George Bataille, *L'érotisme* (Paris: Ed. de Minuit, 1957), Pt, II and III. Cited in Jeanne Parain-Vial, *Tendances nouvelles de la philosophie* (Paris: Ed. du Centurion, 1978) 128.

6 Cf. DTL 139-141; 312 f.,; EPA 206-208.

7 Cf. Deuteronomy 30: 15-20.

8 Cf. The work cited in question 91; the quotation appears on p. 314.

INDEX
OF PROPER NAMES
(NUMBERS REFER TO QUESTIONS)

THEMATIC INDEX
NUMBERS REFER TO QUESTIONS.

Subsidiarity: 82
Suffering: 11
Suicide: 15, 109, 129, 132, 142

Tradition: 91
Technique: 46, 120, 123
Technocrat: 52, 54, 174
Third World: 52, 82f., 86, 96, 99f., 103f., 126, 129
Togo: 92
Tolerance: 61, 62
Torture: 52
Totalitarianism: 11, 51, 64, 75, 106, 139
Transgression: 18, 43, 117
Truth: 51
Tyranny: 44

Ultranaziism: 75
UNESCO: 137
Unhappiness: 6, 10, 12
United Nations: 95, 97f., 102f.
United States: 27, 48, 87, 88, 100, 104
Urchins: 80, 134
USAID: 84, 102

Values, conflict of: 20, 38
Vasectomy: 121
Vietnam: 92, 124
Violence: 27, 30, 135, 143
Vitalism: 32f.
Void, juridical and judicial: 45
Vulnerability: 21

War: 107f.
Weak: 27, 43f., 57 64f.
Wealth, concentration of : 70, 80f., 92, 93, 99, 103-107, 126, 129
Weapons: 131
Welcome: 5, 25, 28, 111-113, 127
West: 58, 103f.
Woman: 5, 14-17, 19-28, 40, 45, 70, 112f., 120-122

Women's liberation: 19
Work: 21, 124
World Bank: 97, 102
World capacity: 92, 139, 140
World Health Organization: 2, 39, 68, 92f., 102
World Order: 102

Youth: 41

Zaire: 92

BIBLIOGRAPHY

Abortion Policies: A Global Review, Department of Economic and Social Development, New York,United Nations: 1992.

Aird, John S., *Foreign Assistance to Coercive Family Planning in China. Response to Recent Population Policy in China* [by Terence Hull] Canberra, 1992.

Anatrella, Tony, *Non à la Société dépressive*, Paris7/24/96: Éd. Flammarion, 1993.

Arendt, Hannah, *Condition de l'homme moderne* [1958], Paris: Éd. Calmann-Lévy, réimpression 1988.

Baudouin, Jean-Louis et Labrusse-Riou, Catherine, *Produire l'homme: de quel droit?Étude juridique et éthique des procréations artificielles*, Paris: PUF, 1987.

Bauer, Peter, *The Development Frontier*, Harvard University Press, 1991.

Bayle, Benoît, *La destruction de l'embryon humain dans la société contemporaine*, Thèse de Doctorat en Médécine, Faculté de Médecine Cochin Port-Royal, Paris, 1992.

Barney, O. (éd.), *Global 2000. The Report to the President*, Arlington, VA: Seven Locks Press, 1991.

Bourget, Vincent, *"Penser l'esclavage aujourd'hui,"* La France Catholique, n. 2328 November 8, 1991, pp 23-25.

Boutin, Christine, *Pour la défense de la vie*, Paris: Éd. Téqui, 1993.

Brunel, Sylvie (éd.), *Tiers-mondes. Controverse et réalités*, Paris: Éd. Economica, 1987.

Camp, L., *The Human Suffering Index*, Population Crisis Committee, Washington, 1987.

Cariou, Pierre, *Pascal et la casuistique*, Paris: PUF, 1993.

Chantel Marie-Magdeleine, *Malaise dans la procréation*, Paris: Éd. Albin Michel, 1993.

Chaunu, Pierre, *Trois millions d'années*, Paris: Éd. Robert Laffont, 1993.

Conly, Shanti, Speidel, J. Joseph and Camp, Sharon L., *U.S. Population Assistance*: *Issues for the 1990s*, Washington, DC: Population Crisis Committee, 1991.

Démographie, dossier in *Défense nationale* Paris, April 1993, 19-74.

Djerassi, Carl, *The Politics of Contraception*, New York and London, Éd. W. W. Norton, 1979.

Dossier avortement: les vrais chiffres, Publication de l'Association pour la Recherche et l'Information démographique (APRD), 12, rue Beccaria, 75012 Paris, 1979.

Dumont, Gérard-François, *Démographie. Analyse des populations et démographie économique*, Paris: Éd. Dunod, 1992.

Dumont, Gérard-François, "Révolutions démographiques," *Le Spectacle du monde*, n.361 April 1992, 80 s.

Dumont, Gérard-François, *La population de la France en 1992*, Paris: APRD, 1993.

Dumont, Gérard-François, "Le vieillissement, un phénomène social majeur," *Revue des DeusMondes*, March 1993, 104-124.

Dumont, Gérard-François, "Avortement: le refus de voir," *L'Homme Nouveau*, April 1993.

Dumont, Gérard-François, *De "l'explosion" à "l'implosion" démographique?*, Communication à l'Académie des Sciences morales et politiques, Paris, October, 18 1993.

Dumont, Gérard-François, "La population mondiale au xx siècle," *Défense nationale*, April 1993, 19-35.

Dumont, Gérard-François, "Démographie et géopolitique," *Défense nationale*, April 1993, 37-54.

Dumont, René, *L'Utopie ou la mort*, Paris: Éd. du Seuil, 1973.

Fonseca Sobrinho, Délcio da, *Estado e População. Uma História do Planejamento familiar no Brasil*, Rio de Janeiro: Ed. Rosa dos Temos et FNUAP, 1993.

Fossion, A., *Passion de Dieu, Passion de l'homme*, Brussels: Éd. A. De Boeck, 1985.

Gallucci, Carlo, "La pillola maldetta," *L'Espresso* (Rome), October 20, 1991, 156-165.

Gauer, Phillippe, *Le choix de l'amour. Diagnostic anténatal*, Paris: Éd. Téqui, 1989.

Gellman, Barton, "Keeping the U.S. First. Pentagon Would Preclude a Rival Superpower," in *New York Times*, March 8, 1992.

Gendreau, Francis (éd.), *Les spectres de Malthus*, Paris: Éd. Études et Documentation Internationales, 1991.

Hancock, Graham, Lords of Poverty. *The Power, Prestige, and Corruption of the International Aid Business*, New York: The Atlantic Monthly Press, 1989.

Hartmann, Betsy, "Population Control as Foreign Policy," *Covert Action* n.39, winter 1991-1992, 26-30.

Hendrickx, Marie, "Quelle mission pour la femme?" in *Louvain* (Louvain-la Neuve), n.4, April 1989, 15 f.

Hennaux, Jean-Marie, *Le droit de l'homme à la vie, de la conception à la naissance*, Brussels, Éd. de l'Institut d'Études Théologiques, 1993.

Herzlich, Guy, "Quand l'Est se 'dépeuple'," *Le Monde* November 9,1993.

Herzlich, Guy, "Le couple population-développement," *Le Monde* December 14,1993.

Inventory of Population Projects in Developing Countries Around the World. 1990-1991, New York: United Nations Population Fund, 1992.

Jasper, William F., *Global Tyranny...Step by Step. The United Nations and the Emerging New World Order*, Appleton, Wisconsin: Western Islands Publishers, 1992.

Jean-Paul II, Encyclique *Veritatis Splendor, La Documentation catholique*, n.2081 November 7, 1993, 901-944.

Kant, Emmanuel, *Fondements de las métaphysique des moeurs*, trans. by Victor Delbos, Paris: Éd. Delagrave, 1959.

Khader, Bicara (ed.), *Le Grand Maghreb et l'Europe. Enjeux et perspectives*, Paris: Publisud, 1992.

Kissinger Report. Implications of Worldwide Population Growth for U.S. Security and Overseas Interests, 1974.

Kojève, Alexandre, *Introduction à la lecture de Hegel*, Paris: Gallimard, 1968.

Kurth, "Hacia el Mundo Posmoderno," *Facetas*, February 1993, 8-13.

La retraite et les retraites, dossier of *Revue des Deux Mondes*, March 1993, 85-124.

Lecaillon, Jean-Didier, "Les démographes se trompent-ils?" *Défense nationale*, April 1993, 67-74.

L'enjeu démographique, Publication de l'Association pour la Recherche et Information démographiques (APRD) 12 rue Beccaria, 75012, Paris, 1981.

Lejeune, Jerome, *L'enceinte concentrationnaire*, Paris: Fayard, 1990.

Lejeune, Jerome and Pouillot, Genevieve, *Maternité san frontières*, Paris: V.A.L., 1986

Lifton, Robert Jay, *Les médecins nazis, Le meutre médical et la psychologie du génocide*, Paris: Robert Laffont, 1989.

Mumford, Stephen D. and Kessel, Elton, "Role of Abortion in Control of Global PopulationGrowth," *Clinics in Obstetrics and Gynaecology* March 13, 1986, 19-31.

Penna Botto, Carlos, "Explosão demografica," *Revista Maritima Brasileira* (Rio de Janeiro) January-March 1993, 103-113.

Perloff, James, *The Shadows of Power. The Council on Foreign Relations and the American Decline*, Appleton, WI: Western Islands, 1990.

Ramond, Janice G., Klein, Renate and Dumble, Lynette J., *RU 486. Misconceptions, Myths and Morals*, Cambridge, MA: Institute on Women and Technology, 1991.

Rawls, John, *A Theory of Justice*, Oxford University Press, 1971.

Reproductive health: a Key to a Brighter Future. Biennial Report 1990-1991. Special 20th Anniversary Issue, Geneva: World health Organization, 1992.

Richman, Sheldon, "Population is no Threat to Progress," *Freedom Daily* (Washington) July 1993, 18-23.

Schwartz, Michael, "Overpopulation and the War on the Poor," Caracas, 1985 (pro manuscripto).

Stanford, Susan M., *Une femme blessée*, Paris: Fayard, 1989.

Torelli, Maurice, *Le médecin et les droits de l'homme*, Paris: berger-Le-vrault, 1983.

Tremblay, E. "Nature et définition de l'acte médical," *Laissez-les vivre*, Brussels: Bruylant, 1982.

Veron, Jacques, *Arithmétique de l'homme*, Paris: Seuil, 1993.

Vilaine, A.M. de, Gavarini, L. and LeCoadic, M. (eds.), *Maternité en mouvement. Les femmes, la reproduction et les hommes de science*, Montreal: Saint-martin, 1986.

Whelan, Robert, *Legal Abortion Examined. 20 years of Abortion Statistics*, London: Spuc Education Research Trust, 1992.

World Population Data Sheet of the Population Reference Bureau, Inc., Washington, 1992.

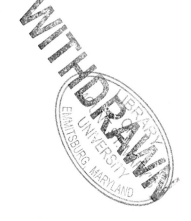